HIV/AIDS in the Middle East and North Africa

HIV/AIDS in the Middle East and North Africa

The Costs of Inaction

Carol Jenkins
David A. Robalino

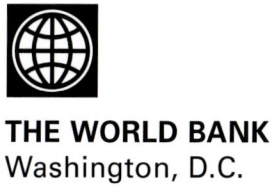

THE WORLD BANK
Washington, D.C.

Contents

Tables

Preface

This volume is the product of a joint exercise among the World Bank, the Joint United Nations Programme on HIV/AIDS (UNAIDS), and the Eastern Mediterranean Office of the World Health Organization (WHO/EMRO). It was produced under the direction of Maryse Pierre-Louis, Lead Public Health Specialist, and Francisca Ayodeji Akala, Public Health Specialist, Middle East and North Africa Region, Human Development Sector, the World Bank (MNSHD); by Carol Jenkins, World Bank consultant and United States Agency for International Development (USAID) Asia/Near East Regional HIV Adviser; and David A. Robalino, Senior Economist, MNSHD, World Bank. Jacques Baudouy, Sector Director, MNSHD, and George Schieber, Principal Economist, Health and Social Protection Manager, MNSHD, provided valuable comments to improve the document. Peer reviewers were Debrework Zewdie, World Bank Global AIDS Adviser; Mead Over, Senior Economist, World Bank Development Economics; Oussama Tawil, Team Leader, UNAIDS Inter-Country Team for MENA, Cairo; and Jihane Tawilah, Regional Adviser, AIDS & Sexually Transmitted Diseases, WHO/EMRO. Henriette Folquet and Darcy Gallucio, Team Assistants, MNSHD, provided support for the presentation of the document.

Because fieldwork was limited, gathering information from credible sources was of utmost importance. After presentation of the main findings of this study at the MENA Regional Public Health Conference in Beirut in June 2002, as well as at the XIV International AIDS Conference in Barcelona, July 2002, a substantial effort was made to update its contents for publication. Between February and May 2003, numerous people helped with this effort. We are particularly grateful to Jihane Tawilah for providing the most recent epidemiological data for the EM Region and to Oussama Tawil for providing up-to-date information on the changing responses in the region and reviewing contents in great detail. In Geneva, Neff Walker (UNAIDS) and Ties Boerma (WHO) responded rapidly to our inquiries.

Country visits, though limited to Djibouti, the Arab Republic of Egypt, Tunisia, and the Republic of Yemen, were invaluable. In those countries several people were particularly helpful. We would like to mention the following:

In Djibouti: Pierre Luigi, World Food Programme; Samira Ali Higo and Michel Etchepare, World Bank consultants; and Dr. A. Sow, WHO.

In Egypt: Dr. Saleh, WHO/EMRO; Dr. Cherif Soliman, Family Health International; Dr. Sussan Bassiri, WHO/EMRO; Wolfgang Schiefer, United Nations Office of Drug Control and Crime Prevention (UNODCCP); Dr. Maha Aladowy, Ford Foundation; Karima Haluf, Population Council; Dr. Alaa Hamed, World Bank; Dr. Nasr el-Sayed, National AIDS Control Programme; and Mark White, USAID.

In Tunisia: Dr. Mourad Ghachem, United Nations Population Fund (UNFPA); Hélène Zoughlami, UNFPA; Dr. Amel Ben Said, Ministry of Public Health; Dr. Zied Latiri, Director of Communication, National Office of the Family and Population, Ministry of Public Health; Elizabeth Bennou, International Planned Parenthood Foundation; Ariel Francais, United Nations Development Programme (UNDP); and Fatma Felah, World Bank.

In Yemen: Amer Majeed Abdul, UNAIDS/UNDP; Dr. Rogers Busulwa, International Cooperation for Development; Hashem Awnallah, World Bank; and Abdul Wahab Anisi, National Centre for Health Education.

Acronyms and Abbreviations

AIDS	Acquired immunodeficiency syndrome
ART	Antiretroviral therapy
AZT	Zidovudine, an antiretroviral drug
BSS	Behavioral surveillance surveys
CBO	Community-based organization
CIS	Commonwealth of Independent States
ELISA	Enzyme-linked immunosorbent assay
EMRO	Eastern Mediterranean Regional Office, WHO
FSW	Female sex worker
GDP	Gross domestic product
GFATM	Global Fund to Fight AIDS, Tuberculosis and Malaria
GNP	Gross national product
HIV	Human immunodeficiency virus
ICDDR, B	International Centre for Diarrhoeal Research, Bangladash
IDP	Internally displaced persons
IDU	Injecting drug user
INGO	International nongovernmental organization
IOM	International Office of Migration
IPPF	International Planned Parenthood Foundation
KAP	Knowledge, attitude, practice
MENA	Middle East and North Africa Region
MNSHD	Middle East and North Africa Region, Human Development Sector, the World Bank
MoH	Ministry of Health
MSM	Men who have sex with men (or males who have sex with males)
MTCT	Mother-to-child transmission
NAP	National AIDS Program
NGO	Nongovernmental organization
PLWHA	People living with HIV and AIDS
pvGDP	Present value of gross domestic product

RTI	Reproductive tract infections
STD	Sexually transmitted disease
STI	Sexually transmitted infection
TB	Tuberculosis
UAE	United Arab Emirates
UNAIDS	Joint United Nations Programme on HIV/AIDS
UNDP	United Nations Development Programme
UNFPA	United Nations Population Fund
UNHCR	United Nations High Commissioner for Refugees
UNICEF	United Nations Children's Fund
UNODC	United Nations Office on Drugs and Crime
UNODCCP	United Nations Office on Drug Control and Crime Prevention (now UNODC)
UNGASS	United Nations General Assembly Special Session on HIV/AIDS
USAID	United States Agency for International Development
VCT	Voluntary counseling and testing
WB	The World Bank
WHO	World Health Organization

Executive Summary

This book reviews the human immunodeficiency virus/acquired immun-odeficiency syndrome (HIV/AIDS) situation in the Middle East, North Africa, and Eastern Mediterranean (MENA/EM) region, and is intended to stimulate discussion and promote dialogue among the region's policy- and decisionmakers. It seeks to provide a framework for multisectoral strategic action to reduce behaviors that risk spreading HIV, to care for and support those who become infected, and to diminish vulnerability among specific segments of society. Although most evidence suggests that overall HIV prevalence is low in the region, greater investments in improved surveillance, prevention, and care are needed now—to main-tain low prevalence levels and preserve the focus on national and regional development goals.

The production of this volume has been a joint effort of the World Bank, the Eastern Mediterranean Regional Office of the World Health Organization (WHO/EMRO), and the Joint United Nations Pro-gramme on HIV/AIDS (UNAIDS). Interviews were conducted with 51 people—including bilateral donors and those in government, U.N. agen-cies, and international nongovernmental organizations (INGOs)—in four countries of the region (the Arab Republic of Egypt, Djibouti, Re-public of Yemen, and Tunisia) and in Geneva between August 18 and September 20, 2001. Newly updated information, as of the beginning of 2003, has been incorporated. Documents were gathered from all perti-nent sources, especially WHO, UNAIDS, U.S. Census Bureau HIV/AIDS Database, and the United Nations Office on Drugs and Crime (UNODC). Because full information for every country in the re-gion was not available from any of these sources, there are inevitable gaps and possible inaccuracies.

Global Experience Responding to HIV/AIDS

In 1991, with the evidence available at the time, experts estimated that 15 million to 20 million adults and 5 million to 10 million children cumulatively would become infected with HIV by 2000. By the end of 2002, UNAIDS/WHO reported that 42 million people were living with HIV/AIDS and 5 million new infections had occurred during the year. The substantial gap between earlier projections and current estimates reflects both the unexpected spread of the virus and the inadequacy of statistics used to track the epidemic. HIV does not always spread rapidly, though it certainly can if conditions permit. Rapid social and economic changes underlie the virus's spread in most of Africa, Russia, Central Asia, Eastern Europe, China, and elsewhere. HIV epidemics have been particularly sensitive to large migrations of people, wars, economic downturns, and other alterations in social stability. UNAIDS/WHO estimates that 1.2 percent of all adults worldwide are currently infected with HIV, and all experts agree that the pandemic's worst effects are yet to come.

Societies cope with HIV and prevent its spread best where governments are open about the issues, provide information and services, and partner with organizations representing affected communities. HIV/AIDS is not simply a pathogen that can be managed with a typical public health approach, and health services alone cannot tackle the breadth of issues that produce vulnerability. A coordinated, multisectoral response is needed that includes appropriate government departments, nongovernmental organizations and community-based groups, bilateral donors, and U.N. agencies.

The collective experience of the past 20 years has shown that the spread of HIV and its effects can be slowed through an approach that reduces risk, vulnerability, and impact as reflected in the U.N. Global Strategy Framework. The highest levels of political commitment are needed to ensure success. The best possible implementation of programs will be achieved with the right mix of policy processes, donor collaboration, and governments working together with civil society actors.

An Opportunity for Prevention: HIV/AIDS Situation in the MENA/EM Region

UNAIDS/WHO estimated that approximately 83,000 people were newly infected with HIV in the MENA/EM region[1] in 2002, and about 0.3 percent of the region's adults are currently infected (UNAIDS/WHO 2002a). Recent evidence suggests that the incidence of sexually transmitted infections, including HIV/AIDS, is increasing, and the total number of AIDS deaths has increased almost sixfold since the early 1990s. In the low- and middle-income countries of the region, HIV/AIDS was the third leading cause of morbidity among people 14 to

44 years old in 1998. Levels of HIV infection among tuberculosis (TB) patients are also rising and, by mid-2001, had reached 26 percent in Djibouti, 4.2 percent in the Islamic Republic of Iran, and 4.8 percent in Oman (WHO/EMRO 2001a). And an alarming rise in HIV continued through 2001–02 among drug injectors in both the Islamic Republic of Iran and Libya.

While these regional figures are relatively low compared with Africa, South and Southeast Asia, and the Caribbean regions, low prevalence does not equate to low risks. Inadequate surveillance methods, which is a universal weakness in the region, can overlook outbreaks in marginalized social groups. Furthermore, *even in low prevalence nations, the situation can change rapidly, as has occurred in Indonesia and Nepal.* Given that HIV/AIDS epidemics tend to exhibit exponential growth, experts expect that the HIV pandemic's worst effects are still to come. *Many countries in the MENA/EM region have enough evidence of risk factors to warrant immediate investments in improved prevention programs.* HIV epidemics are also sensitive to changing economic and social factors, and it is noteworthy that current methods of surveillance in the MENA/EM region will fail to detect meaningful changes where they are most likely to occur. Because the cost of the epidemics to society and economic development can be tremendous, good surveillance and effective prevention programs are relative bargains compared with the cost of epidemics.

Unfortunately, mostly mandatory screening has produced continued low levels of case detection, appropriate behavioral data are lacking, and the region's governments are overconfident in the protective effects of social and cultural conservatism. These factors combined have dictated a low priority for HIV/AIDS. Globally, solid evidence has been amassed that justifies a multisectoral investment in intensified prevention while prevalence is low. Waiting until there is an appreciable rise in prevalence is a costly delay that leads to tremendous human, development, and financial costs. By then, an epidemic may be under way, and it will be too late to prevent the inevitable reductions in human well-being and societal stability, as well as losses in labor productivity, capital investment, and work force availability.

A thorough review of available data exhibits numerous gaps and epidemiological inadequacies. No country, for example, systematically samples and surveys the high-risk groups; instead, the general population, represented by low-risk groups such as antenatal mothers and blood donors, is extensively screened. Although high-prevalence countries can benefit from this type of surveillance, it may fail to record rising rates of HIV among hidden or marginalized groups in a nation thought to have low prevalence. UNAIDS/WHO recommends that *second-generation surveillance*, consisting of targeted HIV serosurveillance, behavioral surveillance, and sexually transmitted infection (STI) surveillance, can reveal the epidemic as it emerges in the most at-risk groups and identify those who are potentially at risk in the immediate future. Instituting this type of surveillance requires considerable collaboration with nongovernmental organizations (NGOs), community groups, and social scientists to gain access to otherwise marginalized groups. But to gain an essential and realistic vision of their national situations, countries must overcome obstacles to collaboration with such groups, and they may require appropriate technical assistance.

Working with the available information, we attempted a rough classification of epidemic type by nation on the basis of the most recent and least ambiguous statistics from the end of 1999 to mid-2001. Overall, despite early cases detected among foreigners and returning migrants, HIV has now begun to spread among citizens in all the region's countries. Patterns are shifting, and a rising proportion of cases are resulting from sexual transmission. These cases may well have been sparked, as demonstrated in Asia (Saidel and others 2003), by earlier clusters of cases among injecting drug users (IDUs), and from them to their sexual partners. Increasingly, infections are occurring in equal proportions of females to males. Djibouti has one of the highest prevalence levels of HIV and has the highest level of sexual transmission. In at least one-half of the countries, significant foci have occurred among IDUs in the past and, in some countries have continued. Other infected groups include males who have sex with males (MSM), sex workers and their clients, prisoners (who are frequently drug users), and patients with sexually transmitted diseases (STDs).

Social and Structural Vulnerability in the Region

Without adequate social and behavioral research, effective HIV prevention programs cannot be planned and carried out. Most published HIV-related research on the MENA/EM region concerns clinical and biomedical issues such as transmission through dialysis. Little substantial HIV-related social or behavioral research has taken place in the region. Designing, implementing, and monitoring prevention programs without information on the sexual and drug-taking behavior of a population and its subgroups is an exercise in failure. Although the expertise exists in most countries of the region to conduct such research, institutional and political support for such research is desperately needed.

Based on the little research available and a variety of other sources of information, we constructed a typology of risk factors. It should be noted that much of this information is unpublished, unscientific, or anecdotal, underscoring the great need for well-conducted research. Simply stated, people are at risk of acquiring an HIV infection because of what they are doing or what they might do if placed in a facilitating situation. We identified two primary groups: an at-risk group and a vulnerable group. In the MENA/EM region, as elsewhere, people with known risky behaviors, such as sex workers, their clients, IDUs, MSM, and those who acquire STDs, are immediately at risk. While it is likely that they represent a minority, any such group can form the core of spread into the rest of the population, depending on the extent and nature of social linkages and networks. Prevention strategies differ considerably for these different groups. The risk factors associated with these subpopulations must be researched and brought to light, if they are to be addressed effectively.

The next group comprises those who may be considered vulnerable, that is, they may be at risk if and when their life situation changes. This group includes, for example, migrants going to work abroad, refugees, mobile workers such as truckers, tourists traveling for fun and recreation, noninjecting drug users who may switch to injecting when the availability or price of the drug changes, and young people in general, in that some proportion will engage in nonmarital sex under certain conditions. An integral part of HIV prevention consists of reducing the vulnerability of people in these social categories. In the MENA/EM region, the HIV-related issues concerning migrants, internally displaced persons (IDP), and refugees are especially significant. Given the large numbers involved in foreign labor migration, AIDS prevention takes on a truly international perspective and must be approached accordingly.

Although a significant number of countries in the region have recorded foci of HIV among IDUs, for example, few countries have made serious attempts to find out how many people are at risk, where they are located, and how to reach them with information and services. In the short run, the perceived negative consequences of public knowledge of such activities may be a valid concern, but in the long run, inaction can adversely affect HIV prevention programs. Learning how to reach at-risk and vulnerable subgroups in discreet, unpublicized ways would contribute significantly to the national AIDS programs throughout the MENA/EM region. This effort will require a special policy process, political commitment, and the creative collaboration of NGOs, social scientists, social workers, and AIDS program managers.

Structural factors, such as poor and dysfunctional health care systems, high rates of unemployment, a lack of access to information and condoms, and inadequate STD and drug-dependency treatment, also increase overall vulnerability. Other structural factors exist as well, including legal restraints on NGOs in some countries or health policies that disadvantage the young and unmarried, the poor, and noncitizens. There is a general lack of policies and legal frameworks for the protection of people living with HIV, particularly in the workplace. In each situation, relevant policies may require review and modification to alleviate barriers to improved prevention and care. The special needs of refugees and others displaced by conflicts must be highlighted in the region. Health authorities cannot ignore the likelihood of spread from migrants, whether legal or illegal, to their local populations.

Macroeconomic Impact

The human cost of HIV/AIDS is incalculable, from the pain and guilt surrounding personal and intimate relationships, to threatened social and political security at the state level. It is nonetheless revealing to examine the costs and losses that *can* be calculated, for these too are great and can have a major impact on a nation's future.

Using the most recently published estimates of HIV prevalence, losses in gross domestic product (GDP) and consumption resulting from the diffusion of HIV/AIDS could be significant in many MENA/EM countries. On the basis of data from nine MENA/EM nations (Algeria, Arab Republic of Egypt, Djibouti, Islamic Republic of Iran, Jordan, Lebanon, Morocco, Republic of Yemen, and Tunisia), calculations for a broad range of diffusion scenarios indicate that the average growth rate of potential GDP could be reduced by 0.2 to 1.5 percent per year for the period 2002–25. The future losses of potential output and consumption during that period could be equivalent to 35 percent of today's GDP, even under conservative assumptions. These losses occur as rising mortality and morbidity reduce labor productivity, capital investments are reduced, and the labor force shrinks.

The analysis also reveals that there could be a considerable impact on health expenditures. By 2015, annual expenditures to treat all AIDS patients may have increased by 1.2 percent of GDP, on average—even with only limited use of antiretroviral drugs. It is possible to find cases in which HIV/AIDS-related expenditures surpass 5 percent of GDP.

Governments have a key role in developing and financing the implementation of policies to confront HIV/AIDS. Indeed, individuals alone cannot devise appropriate mechanisms to contain the epidemic. *To achieve significant results, governments can only intervene if cost-effective interventions are available. Fortunately, international experience shows that low-cost prevention strategies are effective in slowing the spread of HIV/AIDS.* In the case of MENA/EM countries, our analysis shows that increasing condom use and expanding access to safe needles for IDUs can generate savings equivalent to 20 percent of today's GDP. We also show that delaying the implementation of these policies could give rise to accumulated costs for the period 2000–15 that are equivalent to 1.5 percent of today's GDP for each year of delay.

The main messages from these analyses are as follows:

- The risk of an increase in the HIV/AIDS prevalence level in MENA/EM countries is real.

- Expected costs over the next 25 years could be considerable—on the order of 35 percent of current GDP even under conservative assumptions.

- Effective actions can be implemented to prevent the spread of the epidemic, and the costs of these actions would be more than compensated by the savings they generate. and

- *The time to act is today*, when prevalence levels are still low.

Responses

Timing is critical. While national HIV surveillance concentrates on relatively low-risk groups, the virus can reach others. It takes a number of years, particularly in low-prevalence settings, to convince those at risk to alter their behaviors. Where skills are scant and NGOs or community-based agencies have little experience in HIV/AIDS prevention, it takes several years to develop these skills. Finances must be mobilized and efficiently directed, an effort that often requires new administrative structures and mechanisms. Popular, political, business, and religious leaders must be educated to help create an enabling environment in which effective prevention activities can be carried out. Usually, legislative change is required, and legal reform takes time. The MENA/EM region is lagging on most fronts in its defense against HIV.

To date, most decisionmakers in the MENA/EM region have not considered investment in HIV prevention a high priority. Although all countries in the region have National AIDS Committees and 14 of 18 countries have U.N. Theme Groups, their functioning varies considerably. Most countries have instituted actions to ensure safe blood supplies, although this effort is incomplete in some. Efforts to install universal precautions and safe waste management in health services are also inadequate in some countries. Medical management and counseling for people with HIV/AIDS have been set up in many countries, and antiretroviral therapy (ART) is available in several nations. Use of ART to reduce mother-to-child transmission (MTCT) is found less frequently. These measures, however, are only the most basic foundation for a successful HIV/AIDs prevention plan.

Little has been done on the essential work of reducing stigma and discrimination, except among health workers in some countries. Educating the populace about HIV has been spotty and seldom emphasizes the use of condoms for prevention. Condom promotion is nearly absent in the region. High-risk groups are rarely reached with targeted interventions or with systematic surveillance. Harm reduction for IDUs has not been discussed, except in the Islamic Republic of Iran. In general, the region has been slow to respond to the challenges posed by HIV.

HIV epidemics are sensitive to changing economic and social factors and, in the MENA/EM region, current methods of surveillance are unable to detect changes where they are most likely to take place.

The response from U.N. agencies has, until recently, been mainly from WHO/EMRO, which has supported numerous meetings, small studies, and basic program reviews since the 1980s. One or two other agencies have been active in supporting HIV/AIDS prevention in either selected countries or within specific programmatic areas, such as school education. Nearly all other U.N. agencies concur in recognizing that their involvement has been limited to date, but is now changing. UNAIDS has begun funding a series of small activities, mainly through WHO/EMRO, most of which have not yet been evaluated. In general, U.N. agencies have only recently become active in the field of HIV/AIDS in the region.

Few countries have developed an HIV/AIDS policy or strategic national plan that involves all stakeholders, including civil society and groups affected by HIV. Although bilateral donors are present, along with several international and local NGOs, these organizations are inadequately utilized. Only a few nations are demonstrating a commitment to prevention on a scale large enough to make an impact. For example, with funding from the United Nations Population Fund (UNFPA) through a consortium of NGOs, Tunisia has piloted a project for young people that offers appropriate education, counseling and testing, condoms, and STD services. The project has reached about 10 percent of youth and is being scaled up to reach more. In the Islamic Republic of Iran, a large-scale response to rising rates among IDUs has recently been set in motion, including voluntary counseling and testing (VCT), methadone treatment, needle exchanges, and associated activities such as drug demand–reduction programs. Morocco has instituted a large-scale attempt to upgrade STD services and has developed and approved a comprehensive strategic plan. Djibouti is undertaking a similar process, but with its epidemic at a generalized stage, considerable resources will be required to diminish the disease's impact on many citizens and residents. Both the Republic of Yemen and Sudan recently demonstrated public and political concern about HIV/AIDS, a welcome development. During the first two rounds of grants from the Global Fund to Fight AIDS, Tuberculosis and Malaria (GFATM), the Islamic Republic of Iran, Jordan, and Morocco succeeded in acquiring funding.

A Way Forward

The actions urgently needed in each country to respond effectively to HIV/AIDS depend on the stage of the epidemic and other essentially local issues. Recommendations for improving the current situation include:

- Raising the priority given to HIV/AIDS through research, media, and advocacy

- Evaluating what national HIV/AIDS/STD programs have achieved, including proposing ways to strengthen them

- Developing national policy and strategic plans, with associated budgets and the identification of potential resources

- Instituting second-generation surveillance, including STD and behavioral surveys

- Learning to conduct targeted interventions with at-risk groups in a discreet, culturally appropriate manner, in collaboration with NGOs

- Reducing the vulnerability of migrants, IDP, mobile populations, and refugees. This should involve U.N. agencies and appropriate INGOs, and should begin with research to assess situations of risk followed by a process involving all stakeholders to design appropriate and coordinated interventions

- Improving the provision of clear information and means of protection, and taking small steps toward the development of adequate promotion of condoms

- Developing life skills and drug demand–reduction education for youth that is culturally appropriate and effective and recognizes the structural factors associated with drug use

- Reducing vulnerability among youth through multisectoral planning to affect sexual and reproductive health, unemployment rates, educational costs, and information access, among other critical issues

- Ensuring that ART treatment programs are provided and include adequate prevention services as well

- Empowering affected communities by encouraging local NGO development, including increased participation of people living with HIV and AIDS (PLWHA)

- Developing regional networks of experts to fulfill technical needs, while developing local capacity

- Developing programs that are based on sound knowledge of situational context, include increased participation of a wide range of sectors and partners, address vulnerability factors, and have monitoring and evaluation plans and budgets

- Promoting future sustainability of low prevalence through insurance and other health-financing schemes that can help ensure equitable access to health care for people of all socioeconomic strata

- Strengthening country-level information systems in order to monitor and evaluate the situation and response to HIV/AIDS

- Mobilizing additional human and financial resources in support of national responses through collaborative efforts involving a wider range of international, regional, and national partnerships.

These actions will require the collaborative efforts of many partners, including multiple sectors within government, community-based groups, religious and other local leaders, INGOs, bilateral donors, and various U.N. agencies. Most important, the coordination of such a program requires political commitment at the highest levels. If that commitment is attained, the threat that HIV represents to the development goals of the MENA/EM region can be averted. The time to act is today—when the prevalence levels are still low.

Note

1. For the purposes of this book, the MENA/EM region includes Algeria, Arab Republic of Egypt, Bahrain, Djibouti, Islamic Republic of Iran, Iraq, Jordan, Kuwait, Lebanon, Libya, Morocco, Oman, Qatar, Republic of Yemen, Saudi Arabia, Syrian Arab Republic, Tunisia, and United Arab Emirates. Information is included on important neighboring countries that are in the operational region of collaborating U.N. agencies, for example EMRO (Sudan and Somalia) and the United Nations Children's Fund (UNICEF) (Sudan only). West Bank–Gaza (Palestine) has been omitted because of inadequate comparative information.

Introduction

This book reviews the human immunodeficiency virus/acquired immun-odeficiency syndrome (HIV/AIDS) situation in the Middle East, North Africa, and Eastern Mediterranean (MENA/EM) region. It is intended to stimulate discussion and promote dialogue among policy- and deci-sionmakers in the region. It will also provide a framework for multisec-toral strategic action to reduce risk behaviors that spread HIV, to care for and support those who become infected, and to diminish vulnerability among specific segments of society. Although most evidence suggests that overall HIV prevalence is low in the region, intensifying investment in improved surveillance, prevention, and care *now* can ensure the con-tinuation of low prevalence rates and can have a major impact on na-tional and regional development goals.

The production of this volume has been a joint effort of the World Bank, the Eastern Mediterranean Regional Office of the World Health Organization (WHO/EMRO), and the Joint United Nations Pro-gramme on HIV/AIDS (UNAIDS). Interviews were conducted with 51 people—including bilateral donors and those in government, U.N. agen-cies, bilateral donors, and international nongovernmental organizations (INGOs)—in four countries of the region (the Arab Republic of Egypt, Djibouti, Republic of Yemen, and Tunisia) and in Geneva between August 18 and September 20, 2001. Documents were gathered from all pertinent sources, especially WHO, UNAIDS, the U.S. Census Bureau HIV/AIDS Database, and the United Nations Office on Drugs and Crime (UNODC). Because full information for every country in the region was not available from any of these sources, there are inevitable gaps. An up-date with newly available information, as of early 2003, is included.

Chapter 1 briefly reviews world patterns and focuses on experience in low-prevalence countries. Chapter 2 examines available epidemiological data in the region, groups countries in probable epidemic stages, and re-ports on the little information known about the genetic variation of the virus in the region. Chapter 3 develops a typology of risk factors using detailed information gathered in four country visits (Arab Republic of Egypt, Djibouti, Republic of Yemen, and Tunisia) as well as from an extensive bibliography covering all countries in the region.[1] This chapter examines known groups that are practicing risky behavior as well as vulnerable populations who are potentially at risk and explores structural factors contributing to vulnerability. Chapter 4 models the macroeconomic impact of a variety of diffusion scenarios based on the spread of HIV to and from unprotected injecting drug users (IDUs) and sex workers, which are the best understood examples of high-risk groups and are pertinent to specific countries in the region. Chapter 5 reviews the responses to date of health systems, other government sectors, the U.N. and bilateral donors, and other actors in the region. Chapter 6 recommends next steps to improve the current status of programs in the region. The volume concludes with a wide-ranging reference list that was used as background material. Although we extensively reviewed material to prepare this book, it is likely that we were not able to access all existing information at the national level because of time constraints, a limited number of country visits, and, in some cases, difficulty in accessing certain reports.

Note

1. For the purposes of this book, the MENA/EM region includes Algeria, Bahrain, Djibouti, Egypt, Islamic Republic of Iran, Iraq, Jordan, Kuwait, Lebanon, Libya, Morocco, Oman, Qatar, Republic of Yemen, Saudi Arabia, Syrian Arab Republic, Tunisia, and United Arab Emirates. Information is included on important neighboring countries that are in the operational region of collaborating U.N. agencies, for example EMRO (Sudan and Somalia) and the United Nations Children's Fund (UNICEF) (Sudan only). West Bank–Gaza (Palestine) has been omitted because of inadequate comparative information.

CHAPTER 1

Global Experience with HIV/AIDS

In 1991, with the evidence available at the time, experts estimated that by the year 2000, 15 million to 20 million adults and 5 million to 10 million children cumulatively would become infected with HIV (UNAIDS/WHO 2001). By the end of 2002, UNAIDS/WHO reported that 42 million people were living with HIV/AIDS and 5 million new infections had occurred during the year; nearly half of those infections were in females. The worldwide adult prevalence rate had reached 1.2 percent. The great difference between earlier projections and current estimates reflects both the unexpected spread of the virus and the inadequacy of statistics used to track the epidemic. HIV does not always spread rapidly, though it certainly can if conditions permit. Rapid social and economic changes underlie the virus's spread in most of Africa, Russia, Central Asia, Eastern Europe, China, and elsewhere. HIV epidemics have been particularly sensitive to large migrations of people, wars, economic downturns, and other alterations in social stability. Table 1.1 reflects the global situation at the end of 2002.

In 1997, the World Bank developed a classification system for different types of HIV epidemic situations that was widely adopted (World Bank 1999a). The term *nascent* was used as a label for epidemics in which less than 5 percent of people in presumed high-risk groups were infected.[1] This classification system was altered in 1999 by UNAIDS/WHO, which switched to using the term *low prevalence* instead of *nascent* to avoid the connotation that the low levels of HIV prevalence always represented the beginning of a greater epidemic (UNAIDS/WHO 2000a). However, the term *low prevalence* has too often been equated with low priority for national AIDS programs, lending credibility to unsupported notions that little risk or vulnerability exists. UNAIDS/WHO has subsequently promoted *second-generation surveillance*, a combination of HIV and sexually transmitted disease (STD) serosurveillance with behavioral surveillance of the most-at-risk groups, to provide nations with accurate, comprehensive, and forward-looking information about levels of infection as well as levels of risk and vulnerability.

TABLE 1.1

Global Regional Variation in HIV Prevalence, December 2002

Region	HIV/AIDS prevalence among adults (percent)	Adults and children newly infected with HIV	HIV-positive adults who are women (percent)
Sub-Saharan Africa	8.8	3.5 million	58
North Africa and Middle East	0.3	83,000	55
South and Southeast Asia	0.6	700,000	36
East Asia and Pacific	0.1	270,000	24
Latin America	0.6	150,000	30
Caribbean	2.4	60,000	50
Eastern Europe and Central Asia	0.6	250,000	27
Western Europe	0.3	30,000	25
North America	0.6	45,000	20
Australia and New Zealand	0.1	500	7
Total	**1.2 (average)**	**5 million**	**50 (average)**

Source: UNAIDS/WHO 2002a.

Currently, most of the world's countries with generalized epidemics have functional and appropriate surveillance systems of antenatal mothers or other sexually active members of the general population. But countries with low and concentrated epidemics often do not have the surveillance systems needed to track their HIV epidemics properly. This problem clearly exists in the MENA/EM region. No country in the region has set up the type of systematic surveillance of high-risk groups, including their STD and behavioral indicators, required to yield clear information on major risk groups or the effectiveness of AIDS prevention programs (Walker and others 2001). This lack of clear information has led to a lack of visibility, the continued perception of low risk and low priority accompanied by low levels of investment, and, therefore, inadequate levels of protection.

Hidden epidemics in marginalized social groups pose a threat of an expanded epidemic even when repeated testing indicates low prevalence in the general population (Family Health International 2001b). This has happened elsewhere and, based on the scant information available on risk factors, is likely to occur at some time in the MENA/EM region. Figure 1.1 illustrates clearly the progression of the epidemic in Nepal, a progression that took place even as the National AIDS Program continued to monitor the general population. Sentinel surveillance, undertaken semiannually in STD and antenatal clinics throughout the country, showed levels of less than 3 percent and less than 0.1 percent, respectively, as of 1999, but the epidemic continued to grow among groups with whom the surveillance system had little contact. These data illus-

FIGURE 1.1

The Hidden Epidemic in Nepal: HIV Prevalence among Injecting Drug Users and Sex Workers in Kathmandu

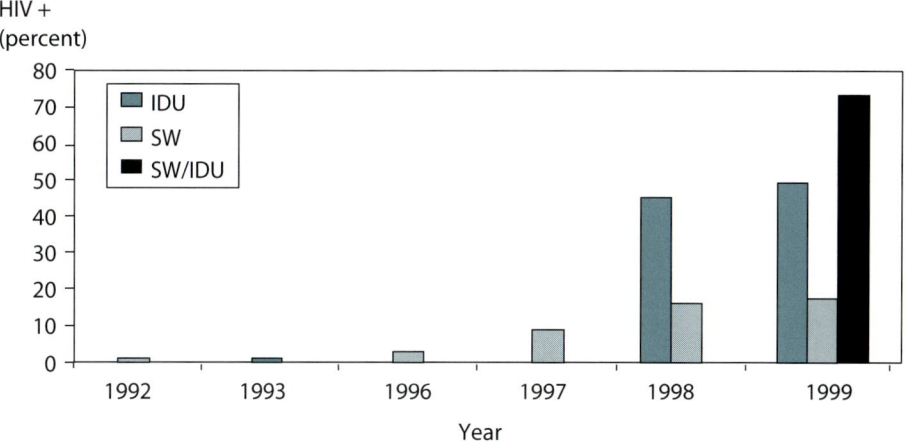

Note: IDU, injecting drug users; SW, sex workers; HIV+ = HIV positive.
Source: Courtesy of J. Ross, Family Health International, Nepal, and United States Agency for International Development (USAID); presented at ICAAP, Melbourne, Australia, Oct. 13, 2001; U.S. Census Bureau 2001.

trate further the intensity of HIV prevalence among unrecognized sub-groups that cross risk zones, for example, the prevalence levels among people who are both IDUs and sex workers is, in this instance, as high as 75 percent.

In Asia, both Nepal and Indonesia have recently experienced expanding epidemics, especially among IDUs (Family Health International 2001a). Advice from experts has for years led these and other similar nations into believing that their epidemics would be self-contained (*The Economist* 2001). Behavioral surveillance, however, has indicated otherwise, showing that IDUs frequently have sexual partners among non-IDUs, including their own wives as well as others. During the past few years, HIV levels have begun to reflect what behavioral studies had revealed earlier. A similar scenario of spread can plausibly be predicted for several countries in the MENA/EM region as well. Significant lessons from elsewhere cannot be ignored (see boxes 1.1 and 1.2).

Where HIV has been allowed to spread, the impact on affected countries has been devastating. In the worst scenarios, teachers die faster than they can be trained, health workers are so often infected that services are crippled or canceled, and farmers can no longer maintain normal agricultural production. The military is almost always affected—often, as in many African countries, to the point that defense functions are seriously hampered. More commonly, military actions taken because of political unrest contribute to the spread of the epidemic. Health and development

---

BOX 1.1

Nepal: Too Little, Too Late

In Nepal, as in almost all other countries in Asia, the first cases of HIV/AIDS were detected during the late 1980s or early 1990s in either a foreign visitor or a returning Nepalese migrant. During the early 1990s, HIV seroprevalence surveys detected HIV infections among STD patients and female sex workers throughout most regions in Nepal. Because of the well-known traffic of both young girls as sex workers and young men as migrant workers between Nepal and India, public health concern focused on the spread of HIV to and from these groups.

IDUs in Nepal were believed to share injection equipment in relatively small and isolated networks and therefore were thought not to pose a threat to the larger society. Surveys undertaken among IDUs in Kathmandu between 1991 and 1994 showed nearly zero prevalence and declining needle-sharing behavior among the men who were in contact with a small pilot needle exchange and education program. But an explosive increase of HIV infections in about one-half of all IDUs occurred during the late 1990s nationally. No other surveillance or study among IDUs took place until 1999, when a national study showed that 40 percent of IDUs nationally were infected with HIV, and more than 50 percent of IDUs in Kathmandu were infected.

A smaller study in Kathmandu seemed to show that those who had been associated with the needle exchange program were less likely to be infected. However, it was clear that the project, while starting early, had not reached a large enough proportion of all IDUs with enough needles to diminish the emerging epidemic. Program expansion was difficult because no policy was in place to support it, and many authorities in the drug control arm of government did not support the harm-reduction approach. It is now too late to avert an IDU epidemic in Nepal. The estimated HIV prevalence in Nepal in 2000 was greater than 50,000 people or close to 0.5 percent of the total 15- to 49-year-old population. A growing proportion of this increased HIV prevalence is the result of injecting drug use, sex work, or a combination of the two.

Source: Family Health International 2001a, 2001b; Karki 2000; Oelrichs and others 2000; Peak and others 1995.

---

gains reflected in increased life expectancy in developing countries are lost, millions of children are orphaned, families' savings and property are lost, and, because of uncontrolled discrimination and stigma, the usual safety nets based on kinship and community support are withdrawn. While both the rich and the poor can acquire HIV, the rich cope more easily. Likewise, both the rich and poor can be vulnerable to HIV, but vulnerability is far greater where people are illiterate, unable to access information and basic services, trapped in unstable survival circumstances,

---

BOX 1.2

Overlooking the Epidemic: The Case of Indonesia

Indonesia is an island republic off the coast of mainland Southeast Asia. As the fourth most populous country in the world with an estimated total population of about 209 million, of which more than 80 percent are Muslim, it is the largest Islamic population in the world. Over the years, Indonesia appeared to have low prevalence, despite projections made in 1994 that it would have 400,000 HIV infections by 1996. "Registered" brothels have existed for more than a century in Indonesia, and sex workers were tested. Even these women showed infection levels of less than 5 percent through 1998. In 1999 and again in 2000, several sentinel sites for female sex workers began to record increasing numbers of HIV infection, with rates from 1.5 percent to 8 percent, and a sample of prisoners reached as high as 17.5 percent. Despite outreach programs, condom social marketing, and mass media campaigns, behavioral surveillance conducted annually between 1996 and 1999 showed that condom use between sex workers and clients did not rise until HIV levels were also rising in 1999.

IDUs were never included in routine serosurveillance in Indonesia. In fact, informally, many people thought there were too few IDUs to bear any significance for an HIV epidemic, and most attention was focused on sex workers. In late 2000, several ad hoc surveys of IDUs throughout Indonesia detected sharply increasing HIV prevalence, up to more than 50 percent in Jakarta. This increasing trend of HIV prevalence can be seen in the blood donor data from the Indonesian Red Cross from 1992 through 2000 in figure 1.2. In recent years, approximately 750,000 to nearly 1 million blood donors have been screened annually for HIV. A marked increase was seen in 1999–2000 and may well reflect the increase among IDUs noted during this same period.

Based on the most recent HIV prevalence findings among different risk groups and on estimates of the size of these groups, a national consensus workshop in Jakarta in March 2001 estimated that there may have been from 80,000 to 120,000 HIV infections in Indonesia in 2000. Indonesia is now classified as a country with a concentrated HIV epidemic primarily among its IDUs, but experience elsewhere indicates that IDUs are not isolated and that the epidemic can easily spread outward to their sexual partners, their children, and others.

Source: Center for Health Research, University of Indonesia 2000; Family Health International 2001a; U.S. Census Bureau 2001.

---

or powerless to alter their situations. Where women have little economic power, they are usually unable to negotiate safety in their sexual relations. Societies cope with HIV and prevent its spread best where governments are open about the issues, provide information and services, and partner with organizations representing affected communities.

FIGURE 1.2

HIV Prevalence in Blood Donors in Indonesia

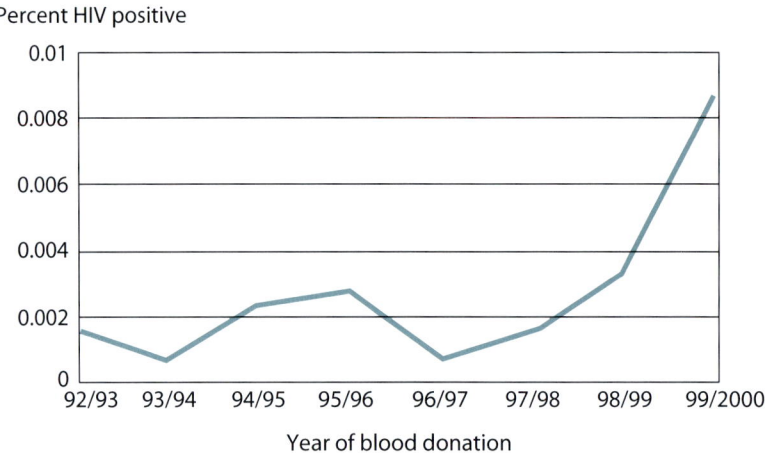

Percent HIV positive

Year of blood donation

Source: Center for Health Research, University of Indonesia 2000.

HIV/AIDS is not simply a pathogen that can be managed with a typical public health approach, and health services alone cannot tackle the breadth of issues producing vulnerability.

The collective experience of the past 20 years has shown that it is feasible to reduce the spread of HIV and its effects through an approach that reduces risk, vulnerability, and impact as reflected in the U.N. Global Strategy Framework (UNAIDS 2001). The highest political commitment is needed to achieve success, with the right mix of policy processes, donor collaboration, and governments working together with civil society to ensure the best possible implementation of programs. Care and support to those already infected and affected are best integrated with prevention programs from the beginning. HIV-infected people and affected communities are powerful advocates and actors when supported positively. No one agency, government or nongovernment, U.N. or bilateral donor agency, can handle the breadth of response necessary. Effective national responses to HIV are consistently hampered by attitudinal barriers to interagency collaboration; bureaucratic inefficiencies; a paucity of skills; fear of social or political repercussions; poor management, including the mishandling of funds; and discriminatory hiring practices. Highly motivated leadership can reduce these factors and discover creative ways to handle the sensitivities involved.

Youth, migrant workers, refugees, traveling businessmen, drug users, and sex workers each have different life conditions. To design HIV prevention programs that are meaningful to people in all these situations, sound social, behavioral, and epidemiological research is essential. In the

MENA/EM region, such research is not only unavailable and frequently considered to be impossible to carry out but also, even when it has been conducted, is often not shared because of intense sensitivities about revealing unacceptable behaviors. The sharing of results of sociobehavioral studies can have a strong and salutary effect on the evolution of HIV/AIDS prevention programs and should be encouraged, at least to a small group of legitimate prevention partners. The Bangladesh experience is illustrative of the effective use of such studies for advocacy (see box 1.3).

BOX 1.3

HIV Behavioral Research in a Conservative Society: Experience in Bangladesh

When, in 1995, the Ford Foundation gave a grant to the International Centre for Diarrhoeal Disease Research, Bangladesh (ICDDR, B) to develop capacity in reproductive health social science research, sexuality research was not even mentioned. Most people at the time did not think such research was possible in Bangladesh, and the research review committee refused to allow any interviews with unmarried people. The program began slowly, and invested a long period in training selected young researchers. Small studies were conducted in a rural area in which ICDDR, B personnel were well-known and appreciated for their programs in diarrhoeal diseases and family planning. These studies examined the terminology and concepts associated with reproductive tract symptoms among men and women. The researchers accumulated terminology used by ordinary people for sexual organs, their functions, and symptoms of disease.

A small study was attempted of clients of brothel sex workers, but it was found that men in rural villages who knew the research team well were more willing to discuss their sex lives. Another small, ethnographic study was conducted of IDUs in a Dhaka slum. In 1997, in cooperation with the Red Crescent Society, an attempt was made to study the sexual behavior of urban young people but, while young men appeared to speak freely, young women were extremely frightened of such discussions. With funding from Family Health International, a large-scale study was conducted of at-risk groups in Chittagong, the nation's largest port. Sailors, fishermen, dockworkers, long-distance truck drivers, as well as both male and female sex workers were interviewed on audiotape, privately and anonymously. This time, more than 600 interviews were acquired, and a deeper understanding was attained of the range of sexual behaviors among these people, the contexts in which these encounters took place, as well as a glimpse into how a hidden sex trade operated in a conservative city. This study eventually led to a large, well-funded intervention on a national scale. Throughout this period, a quietly conducted, in-depth study took place among men who have sex with men (MSM) in Dhaka, using

(Box continues on the following page.)

BOX 1.3 (CONTINUED)

trained men from this community as interviewers. Eventually, even the clients of street sex workers were interviewed in unmarked cars parked on the streets at night.

With this experience, the Social and Behavioral Sciences Program of ICDDR, B agreed to conduct the first national HIV behavioral surveillance surveys (BSS) for the government, in collaboration with laboratory scientists who conducted the serosurveillance. From 1998 to 1999, 3,363 people (IDUs, street and brothel female sex workers (FSWs), MSM, and truckers) were interviewed with a structured questionnaire, but the sampling was not random (except at the brothels) because it was believed to be too difficult to map such groups first in order to acquire a real probability sampling frame. In the following year, with the help of guides from each of the at-risk communities, mapping was accomplished in three cities and true probability samples were attained of 4,449 people (street FSWs, male sex workers, transgender sex workers, brothel sex workers, IDUs, and rickshaw pullers). During these studies, a senior expatriate social scientist served as the Principal Investigator and intensively trained young Bangladeshi researchers. By the third round of surveillance, the Bangladeshi researchers handled an even larger set of probability samples, and full second-generation surveillance was established in the country. The findings of these studies were disseminated to all agencies interested in HIV/AIDS and were instrumental in helping the government decide to make proactive investments in prevention while the nation was still experiencing low prevalence.

Source: Jenkins, Ahmed, and others 2001; Jenkins, Rahman, and others 2001; National AIDS/STD Program, Bangladesh 2001.

Timing is critical. While national HIV surveillance concentrates on relatively low-risk groups, the virus can reach others. It takes a number of years, particularly in low-prevalence settings, to convince those at risk to alter their behaviors. Where skills are scant and nongovernmental organizations (NGOs) or community-based agencies have little experience in HIV/AIDS prevention, it takes several years to develop these skills. Finances must be mobilized and efficiently directed, an effort that often requires new administrative structures and mechanisms. Popular, political, business, and religious leaders must be educated to help create an enabling environment in which effective prevention activities can be carried out. Usually, legislative change is required, and legal reform takes time. The MENA/EM region cannot afford to delay any longer in its defense against HIV.

Note

1. Concentrated = 5 percent or more among high-risk groups; generalized = 5 percent or more within general population, represented by women visiting antenatal clinics, with much higher levels in high-risk groups (World Bank 1999a). UNAIDS/WHO changed the cutoff for generalized epidemics to 1 percent or more in the general population in 2000 (UNAIDS/WHO 2000a).

CHAPTER 2

Review of the HIV/AIDS Situation in the MENA/EM Region

UNAIDS/WHO estimated that approximately 83,000 people were newly infected with HIV in the MENA/EM region in 2002 and that about 0.3 percent of adults in the region are currently infected. Recent evidence suggests that the incidence of sexually transmitted infections (STIs), including HIV/AIDS, is increasing, and that the total number of AIDS deaths has increased almost sixfold since the early 1990s (UNAIDS/MENA 2000; UNAIDS/WHO 2001, 2002a). In the low- and middle-income countries of the region, HIV/AIDS was the third leading cause of morbidity among those 14 to 44 years old in 1998. Levels of HIV infection among tuberculosis (TB) patients are also rising and, by mid-2001, had reached 26 percent in Djibouti (UNAIDS/WHO 2002d), 4.2 percent in the Islamic Republic of Iran (UNAIDS/WHO 2002g), and 4.8 percent in Oman (UNAIDS/WHO 2002m).

While there may be a reluctance to study the often illegal and socially unacceptable behaviors associated with a high risk of acquiring an HIV infection, some national AIDS programs have made efforts to test high-risk groups for HIV. In most cases, these were institutionalized populations (in prisons, detention, or drug treatment centers) and are not likely to be representative of these groups. Because such surveillance has not been conducted systematically, trends cannot be examined, and a hidden epidemic among these groups could be spreading without being detected.

Figure 2.1 compares the rates of AIDS cases per 100,000 people for many countries in the region with a few countries in East Africa. Table 2.1 provides the most recently available official statistics on AIDS as of the end of 2001 in the region, gathered from sources in WHO (EMRO and Geneva), as well as at the country program level. Based on reported AIDS cases to the end of 2001, these figures represent registered cases throughout the region and suggest the levels of transmission taking place 5 to 10 years ago. Such case detection is usually more accurate in countries that have well-functioning health care systems with high coverage of their populations. Reporting of cases is subject to numerous constraints, including the effects of stigma, fear, and ignorance on the part

FIGURE 2.1

Total Reported AIDS Cases per 100,000 People in Selected Countries in the MENA/EM Region, with East African Comparisons

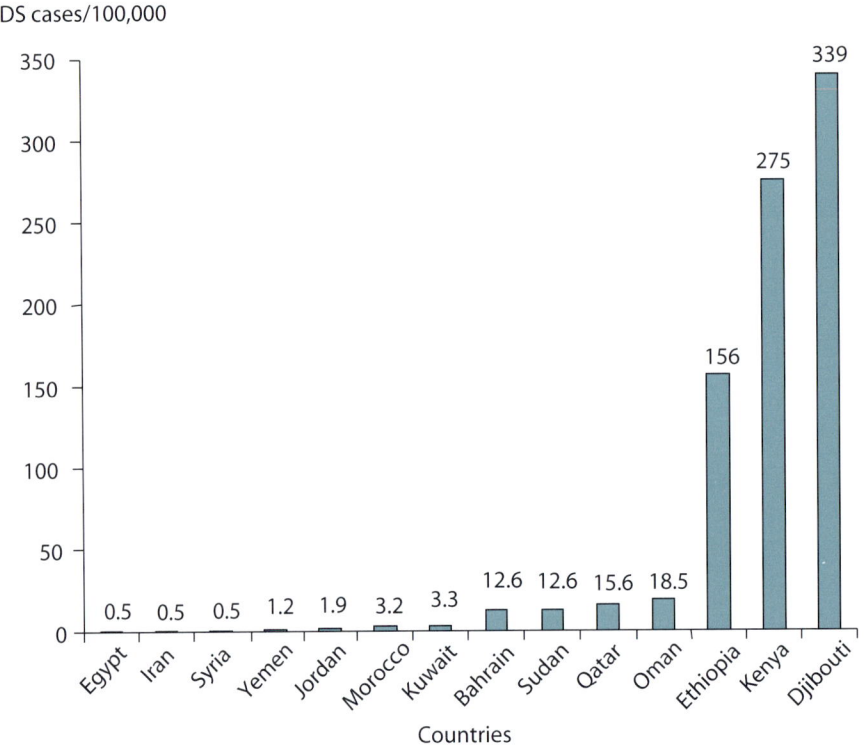

Source: UNAIDS/WHO 2000b, 2002c, 2002d, 2002e, 2002f, 2002g, 2002j, 2002l, 2002m, 2002n, 2002o, 2002p, 2002q, 2002r.

of health professionals regarding diagnosis and the lack of reporting from the private sector. Sometimes expatriates are specifically included (as in Kuwait), and sometimes they are not; in most cases, available data do not clarify this issue. Nonetheless, where other data are scarce, these case reports present a relatively cohesive overview of the region. Djibouti stands out clearly as having a generalized advanced epidemic among other countries in which prevalence remains low or emerging epidemics are concentrated in specific groups. The next most affected countries include Algeria, the Islamic Republic of Iran, Libya, Sudan, and several Gulf states, including Kuwait, Oman, and Qatar. The relatively low levels in all nations but Djibouti must not be considered stable and predictable. History has repeatedly shown that the HIV epidemic shifts in accordance with numerous factors, and only proper serological and behavioral surveillance can detect these changes. AIDS case reporting is capable of detecting past patterns but cannot predict current or future patterns of transmission.

TABLE 2.1

Reported AIDS Cases in the MENA/EM Region, 1987–2001

Country	1987 and before	1988	1989	1990	1991	1992	1993	1994	1995	1996	1997	1998	1999	2000	2001	Total	Population, '000s	Rate per 100,000
Algeria[a]	5	16	17	27	35	34	31	53	32	48	39	49	24	58	17	501	30,841	1.6
Bahrain	1	—	1	2	—	6	3	6	10	11	14	11	9	8	7	89	652	13.6
Djibouti	—	1	6	51	107	144	144	196	231	358	434	111	267	131	—	2,181	644	339.0
Egypt, Arab Rep. of	5	6	9	7	12	23	29	22	16	14	25	33	34	44	42	321	69,080	0.5
Iran, Islamic Rep. of	1	3	5	10	25	16	32	19	16	27	40	21	27	68	76	386	71,369	0.5
Iraq	—	—	—	—	7	6	21	37	16	15	2	4	6	6	4	124	23,584	0.5
Jordan	5	1	6	1	8	7	8	6	2	4	12	11	3	14	10	98	5,051	1.9
Kuwait	1	—	1	1	3	2	2	5	4	5	2	19	4	12	10	71	1,971	3.6
Lebanon[b]	4	3	5	10	13	7	22	12	18	5	8	37	32	21	21	218	3,556	6.1
Libya	—	24	5	11	6	9	2	11	16	21	38	396	72	—	—	611	5,471	11.2
Morocco	10	14	20	26	28	30	44	77	57	66	92	93	165	118	129	969	30,430	3.2
Oman	17	26	26	22	25	32	37	51	28	24	36	24	28	30	35	441	2,622	16.8
Qatar[c]	31	12	9	10	13	5	8	8	6	2	4	3	9	3	2	125	575	21.7
Saudi Arabia	16	6	7	5	10	6	12	38	37	100	112	39	24	24	29	465	21,028	2.2
Somalia	1	4	3	5	—	—	—	—	—	—	—	—	—	73	—	86	5,892	1.5
Sudan	4	64	122	130	188	184	198	201	250	221	270	511	517	652	354	3,866	31,809	12.2
Syrian Arab Rep.	2	2	8	1	7	3	3	4	6	9	8	8	7	7	14	89	16,610	0.5
Tunisia	20	23	19	36	36	38	52	50	65	54	62	44	42	44	48	633	9,562	6.6
United Arab Emirates	0	0	0	8	1	3	1	2	1	2	1	1	2	—	—	22	2,398	0.9
Yemen, Rep. of	0	0	0	1	0	3	4	3	11	60	40	34	34	18	31	239	19,114	1.3

— No data.

a. Algeria is included in the World Bank MENA region but not in the WHO/EMRO region. b. Lebanon's total includes two cases with unknown date of reporting. c. Qatar's total includes four cases with unknown date of reporting.

Source: Al-Jowder 2001; As'ad and Al-Azzeh 2001; Ba-Omer 2001; Egyptian National AIDS Program 2001; El Nakib 2001; WHO/EMRO, personal communication 2003; WHO/EMRO 2001a; Islamic Republic of Iran 2001; Kuwait National AIDS Program 2001; Ministry of Health and Population, Egypt 2001; Ministry of Public Health, Tunisia 2000, 2001; Morocco National AIDS Program 2001; National AIDS Program, Iran 2001; National AIDS Program, Sudan 2001; Sow 2001; Syrian Arab Republic 2001b; United Arab Emirates 2001; Ba-Omer 2002.

In almost all countries, the first case of AIDS was discovered in the middle to late 1980s. Although almost every nation formed a National AIDS Committee and a National AIDS Control Program within a year of having detected the first case, the surveillance systems were largely designed to protect blood supplies and medical services (Bernvil and others 1991; Constantine and others 1990; WHO/EMRO 2001c). In several countries (Arab Republic of Egypt, the Islamic Republic of Iran, Libya, Oman, and Saudi Arabia), outbreaks were detected in hospitals among dialysis patients, cancer patients, and children receiving multiple transfusions for hemophilia or other inherited blood disorders (Aghanashinikar and others 1992; Al-Mahroos and Ebrahim 1995; Al-Owaish and others 2000; Bakir and others 1995; El-Hazmi and Ramia 1989; El-Sayed and others 2000; Hachicha and others 1995; Hassan and others 1994; Hmida and others 1995; Leonard and others 1990; Massenet and Bouh 1997; Watts and others 1993; Yerly and others 2001; Zawawi and others 1997). In most countries, but not all, universal precautions and screened blood supplies have greatly diminished these iatrogenic risks (Daar 1991; Kennedy, O'Reilly, and Mah 1998; Shanks and al-Kalai 1995). Moderate to high levels of hepatitis C in several nations, however, suggests that adequate prevention against iatrogenic transmission of blood-borne viruses does not exist in all medical facilities (Aghanshinikar and others 1992; Al-Mahroos and Ebrahim 1995; Amini and others 1993; Attia 1998; Bakir and others 1995; Benjelloun and others 1996; Cacoub and others 2000; El-Hamzi and Ramia 1989; El-Sayed and others 1996, 2000; Hachicha and others 1995; Kassem and others 2000; Mohamed, al Karawi, and Mesa 1997; Nafeh and others 2001; Groterath and Bless 2002).

Surveillance for HIV infection, as opposed to AIDS case detection, is seriously deficient in the region, as it is only systematic in low-risk groups representing the general population (blood donors, antenatal mothers, and TB patients[1]) and only in some countries. This type of surveillance is not recommended for low-prevalence countries where it is essential to monitor prevalence among those most likely to become infected. Where STD clinics are sentinel sites, at-risk people may be sampled, but there is no information on who they are in a socioeconomic sense, what proportion of those in the community with STDs actually come to those clinics, or if these are the most high-risk people. Standardization of reporting across the region has yet to be achieved. Some nations simply do not report at all some years, while overall poor management of data is evident.

Nonetheless, examining the available data on HIV prevalence reveals a set of different scenarios. Table 2.2 (at the end of the chapter) summarizes the most recent and least ambiguous statistics on HIV available from the end of 1999 to the end of 2002. It lists actual detected HIV/AIDS cases among adult citizens as well as the estimates made by WHO at the end of 1999. Modes of transmission are nearly always calculated on cumulative AIDS cases; if otherwise, this is noted in the table, particularly for recent updates using the last few years only. Where sentinel surveillance has been instituted, it takes place at antenatal, TB, and STD clinics. In Tunisia, a small number (approximately 300) of sex workers are "registered" and, in other nations, the morals police may have access to sex workers, usually by arresting them. No country in the region has access to IDUs outside of treatment centers and the legal and security systems. These systems are often linked. MSM are more likely to be tested through confidential and voluntary services, but this has taken place in only a few countries as small cross-sectional studies (for example, in Egypt and Morocco). Other groups assumed to be at risk who have been tested include soldiers, truck drivers, prisoners, refugees, tea sellers, tourist industry and hotel workers (El-Sayed and others 1996), travelers, noninjecting drug users under treatment or arrest, and taxi drivers. Migration figures prominently in the economic life of the region, and legal out-migrants are nearly always tested before being permitted to work abroad or they are tested in the host country as in-migrants. Many people are tested when they return to their home countries as well. Almost all of this testing is mandatory and without adequate pre- and posttest counseling.

In almost all countries, the first years of testing found most positive results among foreigners, returning citizens, or those infected through blood or blood products. In Lebanon, affected migrants have often been businessmen in trade with or residing in West or Central Africa. In Tunisia, a high proportion of infections were found in IDUs returning from France, where, if caught for drug-related offenses, they are sent home. In Egypt, many were workers returning from the Gulf states. Djibouti has the distinction of being the main port for Ethiopia and also has a large French and, more recently, a U.S. military presence, making it a magnet for sex workers from neighboring countries. Both Djibouti and the Republic of Yemen are hosts to many thousands of Somalian and Ethiopian refugees as well. These conditions may have helped the respective epidemics begin, but cannot be assumed to be the forces that maintain them or that will influence outbreaks in the future.

Need for Second-Generation Surveillance

Surveillance in the region has not yet evolved into second-generation surveillance,[2] including STI and behavioral surveillance, as recommended by WHO. Sampling is not systematic of most high-risk groups, which makes it impossible to examine claims of low prevalence. As seen clearly in the Djibouti material, and corroborated in many other nations, low or absent levels of infection among antenatal women or blood donors can continue for several years while prevalence rises in high-risk groups such as sex workers or IDUs. In several nations, the movement of people at high risk in and out of the country certainly affects the measurement of prevalence. For example, in Djibouti, many thousands of Ethiopians returned to their homes after the conflict with Eritrea subsided. Refugee camps documented in 1996 to have brothel-like conditions for very poor sex workers were nearly empty by 2000 (Tchupo 1998). Under the pressure of law enforcement authorities, shifting patterns of sex work have played a role in the HIV epidemics of several countries. For example, in Thailand and Bangladesh, such pressures have caused sex workers to change locations or venues. Other rapidly changing phenomena include return-migration and refugee flows, as in the Republic of Yemen as a result of political and historical events in the region, and patterns of drug use. Evidence from Asia warns of the rapidity with which noninjecting drug use can shift to injecting drug use (Task Force on HIV and Vulnerability 2000). Repeated monitoring of drug-use patterns has become a necessity in much of the world and is supported by UNODC and WHO using rapid assessment methodology.

Behavioral surveillance of high-risk groups has not begun in the region, with the exception of Djibouti, where such surveys are now under development. Family Health International will be overseeing these surveys as part of an intervention to be carried out by Save the Children (USA) along the road corridor from Mekele in Ethiopia to Djibouti Ville. UNICEF supported an attempt to conduct such studies in Somalia, but it failed to obtain useful information on sexual behavior because of inadequate training of research personnel, among other technical problems. Several nations, such as Djibouti, Egypt, Jordan, Lebanon, Oman, Somalia, Syria, and Tunisia, have determined that their youth are at risk and have carried out surveys of young men and sometimes young women. These surveys cover attitudes and knowledge, but sexual behavior was queried in only a few cases. Among those surveys that did inquire, levels of premarital sex were considerable among males in some countries and very low among females, suggesting that anecdotal accounts of male youth going to commercial sex workers may be accurate. Without information on the sexual behavior of a population as a whole and its subgroups, including nonmarital sexual activities, it is not possible to design, implement, or monitor effective prevention programs.

Conducting both behavioral surveillance and serosurveillance of high-risk groups is dependent on having services to offer, for example, treatment after testing for syphilis. Among hidden populations, developing surveillance means reaching people with services, and, in order to do this, formative documentation of the nature of the drug and sex trade is essential. *In sum, the most important information needed to plan and design HIV/STD prevention programs in the region is lacking.*

Nonetheless, given the information available, one can attempt to classify countries having similar epidemiological profiles into groups (see box 2.1). This classification is based on a combination of the quality and quantity of information accessible and the prevalence levels revealed. The first level is composed of countries that have gathered some information through extensive or repeated testing, albeit not always of the most important groups, and that consistently reveal low levels of transmission. Egypt exemplifies this group; Jordan, Syria, and possibly Saudi Arabia and Iraq also fall into this category. Egypt and Syria do report some information on high-risk groups, but sampling methods and sizes are not always reported; information on the other countries was limited. The second level consists of those countries with a gradually growing accumulation of infections and at least some high-risk groups identified. This second group includes Algeria, Bahrain, the Islamic Republic of Iran, Kuwait, Lebanon, Libya, Morocco, Oman, the Republic of Yemen, Tunisia, and possibly Qatar and the United Arab Emirates (UAE). The third profile is one in which the level of infections appear to be high in the general population. In both Djibouti and Sudan, available data indicate widespread generalized epidemics. A general population survey conducted in Djibouti during 2002 confirmed the presence of a generalized epidemic, but at a lower level of prevalence than previously estimated by UNAIDS/WHO. Somalia is likely to fall into this third category also, though adequate data are lacking.

BOX 2.1

HIV Epidemic Profiles in the MENA/EM Region

Type 1. Repeated testing, consistently low rates, but no consistent, systematic testing (or reporting) of high-risk groups:
- Egypt, Jordan, Syria, and possibly Saudi Arabia and Iraq.

Type 2. Accumulating levels of infection; gradual and slow; some rapid increases in identified high-risk groups:
- Algeria, Bahrain, the Islamic Republic of Iran, Kuwait, Lebanon, Libya, Morocco, Oman, the Republic of Yemen, Tunisia, and possibly Qatar and the UAE.

Type 3. Generalized epidemic levels of HIV:
- Djibouti, Sudan, and probably Somalia.

Viral subtypes have not been identified in all countries of the region, or, if they have, the information has not been published in standard medical journals. However, in Djibouti, subtypes A2, E, and C have been found, indicating sources from West/Central Africa as well as Asia. For viral genetics, see Abid and others 1998; Carr and others 1998; Constantine and others 1990a; Elharti and others 1997; Fox and others 1992; Guman and others 1990; Lasky and others 1997; Mboudjeka and others 1999; Montavon and others 2000; Voevodin and others 1996.

Notes

1. TB patients are often surveyed in low-prevalence countries because they are accessible and because those in charge of TB programs wish to know what proportion of patients is simultaneously infected with HIV. Such patients are to be considered at low risk for HIV, however, as the behaviors associated with acquiring HIV are not factors in becoming infected with TB.

2. Earlier surveillance recommendations were for serology only and did not include behavioral surveillance or STI surveillance. The emerging epidemic scenarios have shown that resources are wasted if they are not targeted at the groups with the most risky behaviors. Second-generation surveillance is the term used to designate an upgraded approach, in which serosurveillance is adjusted for the stage of the epidemic and linked to repeated behavioral surveys.

TABLE 2.2

Profiles of the HIV/AIDS Epidemics in Countries of the MENA/EM Region

Country	Date of first recorded AIDS case	Estimated adult prevalence level (percent) (UNAIDS/WHO)	Adults and children living with HIV/AIDS (reported [r] and estimated [e] by UNAIDS/WHO, end 2001)	Female reported AIDS cases or reported HIV infections (percent)	HIV in high-risk groups (percent)	Features of epidemic transmission modes among reported AIDS cases, 1997–2001; HIV prevalence in general population; major risks; indicators of change
Algeria	1985	0.1	1,067 (1/01) [r]; 13,000 (adults) [e]	27 (AIDS)	1.2 in FSWs (1988). 10 in 20 FSWs (2000); 3 in 139 FSWs (2000); STD clinics at 6 sites, 1.3 at Tamanrasset, 4 at Oran, rest zero (2000)	41% heterosexual, 5% homosexual, 18% IDU, 10% blood, 2% MTCT, <1 other, 24% unknown; 0.9% HIV prevalence at 4 antenatal sites (2000); 0.3% in 345 TB patients (1998); 0.4 in 1,984 antenatal mothers ('00); high levels of migrants from West and Central Africa transiting through southern area; FSWs from Algeria and elsewhere.
Bahrain	1985	0.3	216 (December 2000 [r]); <1,000 [e]	7 (AIDS); 11 (HIV, July 2001)	1.6 in 242 multitransfused children with hemolytic anemias (1995); 0.3 in 291 IDUs (2000); 0.9–2.3 in IDUs (1998).	11% heterosexual, 4% homosexual/bisexual; 72% IDU, 2.4% MTCT, 10% blood; 67% all cases in IDUs (2001); 0 in 2,079 blood donors (1999); 0.2 in 627 antenatal women (1998); migrant sex trade, opiates.
Djibouti	1986	2.8	3,500–14,500 [e] (1999)	21 (AIDS, 1997–98); 54 among 15- to 29-year-old cohort.	22 in STD patients (1996); 28 in FSWs (1998); >50 in street sex workers and 26 in bar sex workers (1996).	99% heterosexual, 1% MTCT (1997–98); 1.9% in private antenatal clinic (1999); 26% in TB patients (2001); 1.8%–3.1% in blood donors (2000); STDs: 3.2% syphilis in antenatal mothers (1997); in 2002, general population 2.8% (95% CI 1.2% to 4.5%, 1999); high levels of commercial sex, refugees.
Egypt, Arab Rep. of	1986	<0.1	1,291 (June 2002) cumulative [r]; 8,000 [e]	11; 17.3 (NAP)	1 in 102 MSM (1999); 0.79 in 382 MSM (2000); 0.86 in 815 MSM (2001); 0 in 129 FSW (2001); 0 in 920 STD patients (2001).	45% heterosexual, 21% homosexual, 6% IDU, 16% blood, <1% MTCT, 11% unknown; 0.006% in blood donors (2000); 0 antenatal: 0.6% in TB patients; 75% infections acquired in Egypt.
Iran, Islamic Rep. of	1986	<0.1	20,000 [e]	8	0.72 in 140,277 drug users tested over time; 0.5 in 8,202 IDUs (1998); 2.3% among prisoners, mostly drug users, in 2000; 0 in 5,700 STD patients (1998); 0 in 1,605 FSWs (1998).	10% sexual; 64% IDU, 6% blood, 1% MTCT, 19% unknown; 4.2% in TB patients (2000); rapid threefold increase in HIV/AIDS in 2001; 4% among VCT center users (2001); sex work, polygamy also risk factors.

(Table continues on the following page.)

TABLE 2.2 (continued)

Country	Date of first recorded AIDS case	Estimated adult prevalence level (percent) (UNAIDS/WHO)	Adults and children living with HIV/AIDS (reported [r] and estimated [e] by UNAIDS/WHO, end 2001)	Female reported AIDS cases or reported HIV infections (percent)	HIV in high-risk groups (percent)	Features of epidemic transmission modes among reported AIDS cases, 1997–2001; HIV prevalence in general population; major risks; indicators of change
Iraq	1991	< 0.1	<1,000 [e]	9	Mandatory screening for prisoners, STD patients, health and hotel workers; premarital tests; etc.	93% heterosexual, 86.1% blood, 4.6% MTCT (1999); STDs: reported cases increased between 1999 and 2000; 0.1% syphilis and 0 HIV in pregnant women (2000).
Jordan	1986	<0.1	118 (June 2001) [r]; <1,000 [e]	13 (AIDS); 26 (NAP)	No surveillance except prisoners; none infected of 945 tested (2000).	40% heterosexual, 3.2% homosexual, 3.2% IDU, 38.9% blood, (1997–2000), 1.1% MTCT, 13.7% unknown; only 1/281 TB patients infected; 0.03% among blood donors; none among antenatal mothers tested 1992, 1994, 1999; KAP study (1999) of 3,200 people revealed 4%–16% sex outside of marriage in last year, of which 10% MSM.
Kuwait (includes expatriates)	1984	0.12	835 (December 2000) [r]; 1,300 [e]	18	0 in 2,600 STD patients; mandatory testing for sexual offense prisoners, IDUs in treatment/custody; 0 in 193 IDUs (2000).	73% heterosexual, 6% homosexual, 6% IDUs; 2% MTCT; 6% blood, 8% unknown; 275,307 people screened in 2000, 1.7% HIV positive; 0 in pregnant women; STDs: increased from 1,002 in 1991 to 6,043 in 1997; 30% gonorrhea, 1.6% syphilis; HIV types B & C, via India; migrants/sex/heroin.
Lebanon	1984	0.09	613 (December 2000) [r]; 1,500 [e]	16 (AIDS); 21 (December 1999 HIV/AIDS cases)	In 1999, 0 infected of 205 select FSWs; 0.2 in prisoners; 6.3 of all reported HIV cases are IDUs, all males.	47% heterosexual, 28% homosexual, 3% IDUs, 15.6% blood, 6.7% MTCT (cumulative); >50% recent cases local origin; rising percentage of women; general population behavioral surveys in 1991 and 1996 show drop in ever use of condom from 40% to 33%.
Libya	1990	0.2	611 (1999) [r]; 1,182 (end 2000) [r]; 7,000 [e]	—	571 new infections in 2000, 98 among IDUs.	56% heterosexual, 22% blood, 22% MTCT (cumulative, but not currently accurate; outbreaks in hospitals from lack of infection control, 370 children in 1998; 22% in blood donors (1998); 0.3% in 296 TB patients (1998).

Country	Year	Rate	Number			Notes
Morocco (includes expatriates)	1986	0.1	809 (September 2000) [r]; 13,000 [e]	36:50 (among new cases)	0.16 in STD patients (2000); no surveillance among FSWs or MSM.	70% heterosexual, 9% homosexual, 6% IDUs, 3% blood, 2% MTCT, 6% other, 4% unknown; <1% in antenatal women (2001); rising rates in some areas, Tangiers higher in IDUs, Marrakech higher in MSM. 94% of all cases among Moroccans.
Oman	1987	0.1	600 (February 2001) [r]; 1,300 [e]	32	In 1999, 5 in 135 arrested IDUs; 8.3 among 60 IDUs (2000); 0 HIV in 337 STD patients (2001).	41% heterosexual, 11% homosexual, 2% IDUs, 22% blood, 6% MTCT, 2% other, 17% unknown; 2% in TB patients (2000); STDs: incidence rate of reported cases dropped from 92 to 48.6 per 100,000 between 1996 and 2000; among 245 men in social clubs, 13% nonmarital sex in past year (1995).
Qatar	—	0.09	300 [e]	29 (cumulative AIDS)	In 1999, 5 in 2,249 STD patients.	20% heterosexual, 4.8% homosexual, 58% blood, 8% MTCT, 9.6% unknown; 0 in 2,464 blood donors (1999).
Saudi Arabia	—	—	—	34 (AIDS 1997–98); Two-thirds of AIDS cases among male expatriates.	2.3 in multitransfused children (1989); 0.14 in 2,102 IDUs (1997).	72% heterosexual, 6% homosexual, 2% IDUs, 15% blood, 4% MTCT (1997–98).
Somalia	1987	1.0	43,000 adults [e]	—	2 to 4 in FSW (1990)	Little information, MTCT 3%; 3%–9% in antenatal mothers (2000); blood donors range from 0.8% to 4.4%; 6.9% in 649 TB patients (1999).
Sudan	1985	1.6	450,000 [e]	29.8 (AIDS)	1 in out-migrants, 4.3 among 470 refugees, 4.4 among sex workers, 2.5 among tea sellers, 1.6 among TB patients (2002).	97% heterosexual, 3% MTCT (1997–2001), 1.4% HIV in blood donors (2000); 1%–5% antenatal clinics, 7.7%–20% TB patients; clear rise starting late 1980s, generalized by mid-1990s; STDs: 2% syphilis in antenatal mothers, 9% in STD patients (2001); national survey n = 7,385, 1.6% (2002).
Syrian Arab Rep.	1987	0.01	145 (July 1999, NAP)	21 (July 1999, NAP)	As of 1998, STD patients 0.12; FSWs 0.12; bar girls 0.04; MSM 0.59; 0 in IDUs.	73% heterosexual, 8% homosexual, 8% IDUs, 8% blood, 4% MTCT (1997–2000); 250,000 people tested yearly, almost all mandatory; 0.0015% in blood donors, 0.005% in Syrian travelers before departure; few cases detected; STDs: April to June 1999, 2,342 cases reported at four centers according to syndromic method.

(Table continues on the following page.)

TABLE 2.2 (continued)

Country	Date of first recorded AIDS case	Estimated adult prevalence level (percent) (UNAIDS/WHO)	Adults and children living with HIV/AIDS (reported [r] and estimated [e] by UNAIDS/WHO, end 2001)	Female reported AIDS cases or reported HIV infections (percent)	HIV in high-risk groups (percent)	Features of epidemic transmission modes among reported AIDS cases,1997–2001; HIV prevalence in general population; major risks; indicators of change
Tunisia (includes expatriates)	1985	0.06 (March 2001)	985 (December 2000) [r]; 2,200 [e]	40 (AIDS, 1998–99)	0 to <1 in registered FSWs throughout 1990s; 0 in 570 FSWs (1999), 0.22 in 458 FSWs (2001).	51% heterosexual, 10% homosexual, 27% IDUs, 8% blood, 4% MTCT (1998–99); 0 in 108 antenatal mothers (1999); >50% detected as AIDS; all infected females and 30% males acquired infection in Tunisia; high proportion among expatriates; 0.25% in TB patients (1996); 0.003% in blood donors.
United Arab Emirates		0.18	2,300 (January 2000) [e]	—	—	—
Yemen, Rep. of	1990	0.01	960 (December 2000) [r]; 9,900 [e]	33 (2000); ~50 HIV (2000)	5 in 88 FSWs (1998); 3 in 585 STD patients (1998); 27 in 147 prisoners (1998); 2.7 in FSWs (1999); 7 in FSWs (2001); 1.8 in 284 STD patients (2000).	77.3% heterosexual, 15.9% homosexual, 6.8% blood (1998); more than 50% infections acquired in Republic of Yemen; gender ratio changed from 4:1 (male to female) in 1995 to 2:1 in 1999 and 1:1 in 2000; 0.7% in 11,070 "low- risk" people (1998); 0.04% in 19,813 blood donors (1998) rose to 0.28% in 2000; 6.9% in TB patients (1999); 45% HIV infections among Yemenis.

—Not available.

Note: Proportions represent AIDS cases and assumed modes of transmission according to WHO 2001. CI, confidence interval; FSW, female sex worker; IDU, injecting drug user; KAP, knowledge, attitude, practice; MTCT, mother-to-child transmission; NAP, National AIDS Program; STD, sexually transmitted disease; TB, tuberculosis; VCT, voluntary counseling and testing.

Source: Abdelmajid 1999; Al-Jowder 2001; Al-Owaish and others 2000; As'ad and Al-Azzeh 2001; Ba-Omer 2001; Ben Said 2001a, 2001b; Bouakaz 1998; Bouakaz 2000; Egyptian National AIDS Program 2001; El Nakib 2001; WHO/EMRO 1995, 2000a; 2001a; El-Sayed 2002; Etchepare 2001, 2002; Family Health International 2001c; Farza 2001; Hermez 2002; Islamic Republic of Iran 2001; Kuwait National AIDS Program 2001; Ministry of Health, Djibouti 2001; Ministry of Health in collaboration with UNAIDS and WHO, Jordan 1999; Ministry of Health and Population, Egypt 2001; Ministry of Public Health, Tunisia 2000, 2001; Morocco National AIDS Program 2001; Mosbah and Ben Yahi 1998; National AIDS Program, Iran 2001; National AIDS Program, Sudan 2001; Njoh and Zimmo 1997; Preble 1996; République Algérienne Démocratique et Populaire Ministère de la Santé et de la Population/Direction de la Prévention/Institut National de Santé Publique 2000; Rosa 1999; Sow 2001; Sudan National AIDS Control Program 2000, 2001, 2002; Syrian Arab Republic 2001a; Tchupo 1998; UNAIDS/WHO 2002a, 2002b, 2002c, 2002d, 2002e, 2002g, 2002h, 2002i, 2002j, 2002k, 2002l, 2002m, 2002n, 2002o, 2002p, 2002q, 2002r, 2002s, 2002t.

CHAPTER 3

A Typology of Risk Factors

The lack of solid epidemiological and sociological understanding of the contexts and determinants of risk behaviors throughout the region seriously limits intervention strategies. In the interest of facilitating a discussion concerned with devising new and creative means to implement properly targeted prevention programs, the following section examines the presumed main risk factors in the region and attempts to examine selected social, economic, and structural factors that can influence vulnerability.

At-Risk Groups

Simply stated, people are at risk of acquiring an HIV infection because of what they are doing or what they might do if placed in a facilitating situation. The first group constitutes those who currently have multiple, concurrent (within the past year) sex partners or inject drugs; the second group consists of all those whose lives may place them in situations in which these behaviors are more likely, for example, migration away from home, particularly when under insecure conditions.[1] A common situation of vulnerability is when noninjecting drug use shifts to injecting drug use because of changes in availability and price of drugs. Prevention strategies differ considerably for these different groups. In the MENA/EM region, there is evidence of immediate high risk for the following groups: IDUs, sex workers, their clients, and MSM.

Few countries in the region have made serious attempts to find out how many of these people are at risk, where they are located, and how they may be accessed for education and services. In the short run, potential negative consequences of public knowledge of such activities may be a valid concern in many circumstances, but in the long run, lack of knowledge can seriously impair planning and design of HIV prevention programs. Learning how to reach these people in quiet and unpublicized ways would make a great contribution to the National AIDS Programs throughout the MENA/EM region. This effort will require a special policy process, political commitment, and the creative collaboration of NGOs, social scientists and social workers, and HIV/AIDS program managers.

Injecting Drug Users

The UNODC reports that drug-trafficking routes have been shifting in the eastern Mediterranean and parts of northern Africa in recent years. In addition to the well-known opium and heroin traffic from Afghanistan to the Islamic Republic of Iran, a major transit route through Turkey and neighboring countries provides heroin and stimulants to the markets of the Gulf states. In addition, illicit drugs are smuggled into the Arabian peninsula from southwest Asia, and synthetic drugs are produced in some countries of the region. As elsewhere, changing drug-trafficking routes produce localized changes in patterns of drug consumption along those routes. Social change and the long-term consequences of the drawn-out conflicts that are characteristic of the region may also have an impact on drug use (Toufic 1996–97). Most countries in the MENA region report data that point to increasing drug use, especially among young people, mainly of cannabis, heroin, and stimulants, including large-scale use of fenetylline. Strong cultural and social stigma is likely to deter users from admitting to their addictions and seeking help (UNODC 2003). Coupled with inadequate HIV surveillance as well as a real paucity of information on the drug trade and drug-use patterns, it is clearly possible that hidden HIV epidemics among drug users are to be found throughout the region.

A significant number of countries in the region has recorded foci of HIV among IDUs. Recent outbreaks have been documented in Bahrain, the Islamic Republic of Iran, and Libya and concentrations of infections have been reported in Algeria, Egypt, Kuwait, Morocco, Oman, and Tunisia. To a lesser extent, Jordan, Lebanon, Qatar, Saudi Arabia, and Syria have also reported such clusters of cases. No information was available on the UAE or the Republic of Yemen, although in the Republic of Yemen there is some acknowledgment of the potential for IDU transmission. In 1998, IDUs represented two-thirds of all cases of AIDS reported in Bahrain and half of all cases reported in the Islamic Republic of Iran. In the same year, IDUs represented 30 percent of all recorded HIV (not yet AIDS) cases in the Islamic Republic of Iran, rising to about 65 percent by 2001. In one study in 1991, 242 IDUs under treatment in Manama, Bahrain, had an HIV prevalence of 21.1 percent (Al-Haddad and others 1994; WHO/EMRO and UNAIDS 2001), though subsequent studies revealed much lower levels. Oman reported a level of 5 percent HIV among IDUs tested in custody in 1999 (WHO/EMRO and UNAIDS 2001). Morocco reports 7 percent of all cumulative AIDS cases among IDUs (Morocco National AIDS Program 2001).

In these countries, IDUs were tested when in contact with authorities, either after arrest or in treatment facilities. Although about one-third of reported AIDS cases were among IDUs in Tunisia, it is thought that they all acquired their infections when outside of the country. Because of the strict prosecution of illegal drug users in most countries of the region, access to out-of-treatment IDUs is difficult, and sentinel surveillance of street-level IDUs has not been possible. Hence, the bias in prevalence levels cited is unknown. Most estimates are based on analysis of cumulative reported AIDS cases.

With the exception of Egypt (United Nations Office of Drug Control and Crime Prevention [UNODCCP] 2001b, 2001c), the Islamic Republic of Iran (Razzaghi and others 1999), Lebanon (Ingold and the Lebanese Research Cooperative 1994), and Morocco, to our knowledge, there have been no rapid assessments or other studies to establish the profile of IDUs in each country. Even where such assessments have taken place, these can become outdated quickly as drug-use patterns can shift rapidly and remain hidden. The 1994 assessment in Beirut estimated that 10 percent of all users were IDUs and 40 percent of these IDUs shared needles. In Egypt, several studies suggest that injecting poses a possible serious problem, although better sampling is required in order to be certain (see box 3.1). In Jordan, it is said that there has been a recent shift from use of hashish to the use of injectable heroin, cocaine, and opium (UNODCCP 2000c). In Kuwait, according to local press reports, there are more than 29,000 drug addicts in a population of 1.7 million (Reuters 2001a; Whitaker 2000). Although heroin and opium are reportedly in use, no estimates were found of the proportion of users who are injecting. Libya is estimated to have about 7,000 drug users, most of whom inject heroin. Almost all (564) of the 571 new HIV infections reported in Libya during 2000 were among drug users (UNAIDS/WHO 2002k).

In the Islamic Republic of Iran, the situation among IDUs is better understood than elsewhere (Aqaie 2001; Arbesser, Bashiribod, and Sixl 1987; *Iran Daily* 2001b; Islamic Republic of Iran 2001; Moore 2001; Muir 2002; National AIDS Program, Iran 2001; Razzaghi and others 1999). The first real outbreaks were seen in 1991 in prisoners, most of whom were arrested for illegal drug use. Little evidence of HIV was found again until 1996, when 29 percent of injectors in two prisons were found to be infected. By 2001, 10 prisons had reported HIV infection among injectors, with one site as high as 63 percent. IDUs under treatment have lower prevalence levels, which were recorded recently at 12 percent, indicating a high probability of transmission taking place in prisons.

BOX 3.1

Injecting Drug Users in Egypt

In Egypt, more information is available on drug-related risk for HIV infection than on sexual behavior–related risk. Since the mid-1990s at least three key studies have supported the need for considerable HIV prevention efforts among drug users. The first study revealed that 6 percent of 16,645 young people in five governorates had used illicit drugs at some time in their lives. The second study, a situation assessment conducted by the Ministry of Public Health and UNODC in five governorates (n = 697) found that 16.4 percent of a sample of 175 drug users reported injecting. Injecting was most common in Cairo, followed by Sinai. The drugs injected were heroin and psychotropic medicines, often purchased as tablets and crushed. These IDUs were more often older, single, skilled laborers and had higher incomes than other drug users. Sexual orientation was queried among all drug users; 1.1 percent were homosexual and 2.2 percent were bisexual.

The third, most recent study, of those in drug-treatment centers (n = 152) found that 41 percent were IDUs. The sharing of equipment and unsafe sexual practices were both reported as risks for HIV. These studies point to the great need for reaching drug users outside of treatment through outreach in order to provide suitable programs for treatment, education, and HIV testing.

Source: El-Sayed 2002; UNODCCP 2001b, 2001c.

A rapid assessment by Razzaghi and others (1999) was carried out in the Islamic Republic of Iran in 1998 under the guidance of the UNODCCP (now UNODC). This well-executed study showed that heroin and opium use was widespread, with about 2 percent of the population using these drugs, a level comparable to that in Russia and many times greater than in the United States. An estimated 10 percent to 18 percent were currently injecting, for an estimate of about 200,000 IDUs. More than 90 percent were men, but women were probably underrepresented. Among men, the mean age at onset of illicit drug use was 22 years old ± 7 years. About one-half the men were married, and one-third of these reported having had extramarital sex, mostly with sex workers. About 70 percent of the unmarried men were also sexually active, 74 percent with sex workers and 30 percent with other men. The assessment also showed the serious lack of HIV prevention among IDUs and the inadequacies in treatment programs. Since that time, the Islamic Republic of Iran has attempted to expand and improve treatment options, including trials with methadone, and has begun harm-reduction programs that include needle exchanges (U.S. Census Bureau 2001; Yeghaneh 2001). Recent studies confirm widespread injecting drug use by prisoners. The Islamic Republic of Iran's national organizations have actively responded to the well-documented serious risk of HIV transmission in their nation and have begun to examine issues surrounding sex work as well (Dareini 2001; Reuters 2001b).

Similarly well-conducted studies have not yet taken place in most other countries. Coupled with the fact that at least nine other countries have recorded a significant number of infections among IDUs, the lack of data on this issue reveals widespread ambivalence about drug use in the region. In 1999, WHO/EMRO organized an intercountry consultation on demand reduction in which most countries reported having a mixed policy, treating the drug addict as both a criminal and a patient (WHO/ EMRO 1999). There are few treatment facilities; they are generally based on detoxification and often do not have programs to prevent relapse upon release. Methadone or other substitution treatment is not commonly available. Harm reduction to diminish the spread of HIV or other blood-borne infections in prisons has not been considered except in the Islamic Republic of Iran, but may be needed in several countries.

Sex Workers

Women and sometimes men engage in commercial sex throughout the world, and the MENA/EM region is no exception. Religious principles, social pressures, and, in some instances, punishments are strong and keep the various types of sex trade hidden. Nonetheless, numerous reports point to the high-risk situation surrounding sex workers in many countries in the region. The best documentation regarding sex work in the region comes from Djibouti, where the trade is far less hidden than elsewhere (Constantine and others 1989, 1992; Couzineau and others 1991; Etchepare 2001; Fox and others 1988, 1989a, 1989b; Philippon and others 1997; Rodier and others 1993a, 1993b; Tchupo 1998). Previously, women from neighboring countries dominated the trade, but, of late, Djibouti women are increasingly involved. In 1998, a brief assessment of the STI situation in Djibouti described several levels of sex work. Starting with relatively highly paid women accessible at five-star hotels serving the wealthy, foreigners and Djibouti nationals alike, the list works its way down to street children sex workers and brothel-like scenes for women in refugee quarters that are reportedly now mostly abandoned. In between, there are bar and restaurant workers serving the military; street workers providing "quick" sex, mainly to Djibouti men at various sites around town; as well as *geeza* women (Somalian) who serve where men chew *qat* (Tchupo 1998). Reaching these many different women would require customized strategies. Collected epidemiological material shows distinctly different rates of HIV among bar girls or hostesses compared with street sex workers (see figure 3.1). In Djibouti, bar girls have been checked and offered STI services by French army authorities as a matter of prophylaxis for many years.

Algeria, Lebanon, Morocco, Tunisia, and Syria also have data on HIV among sex workers. Tunisia has a tradition of registering sex workers, but these number only about 300, and many more are thought to be in the clandestine trade. In Sana'a, Republic of Yemen, sex workers frequent known streets, working in a system in which rooms can be rented in apartments of women who participate in the network. It is thought that many of these women are from neighboring African countries. One recent report states that HIV prevalence among arrested sex workers in the Republic of Yemen reached 7 percent (Al-Qadhi 2001). Other countries have locales, some more hidden than others, to which it is reported that women from a variety of countries, particularly South and Southeast Asia, are recruited (Blanchet 2002). Egypt has its "red flats," rental spaces kept especially for this activity (El-Gawhary 1995). Street-based and other forms of sex work have been documented in writings about Cairo over recent years. Higher-paid "call girls" operate in better hotels in many countries. Because of the great need for keeping the business hidden, cell-phone-carrying brokers play a major role, and most appear to be female. Sex work is increasingly being openly recognized as a social issue in the Islamic Republic of Iran and Lebanon. Concern has been expressed in the Islamic Republic of Iran about the potential for temporary marriage, known as *sigheh* or *muta'a*, to contribute to the spread of HIV (Haeri n.d.; Heise, Moore, and Toubia 1996). Bahrain and the Islamic Republic of Iran have also attempted to tackle the trafficking of women as sex workers (Reuters 2001a, 2001b).

Hardly any in-depth studies have been made on commercial sex in the MENA/EM region, and some of the information reported in this book is based on unconfirmed discussions with local people. The main clients of sex workers have not been identified. Clearly, however, adequate data, such as increasing rates among STD patients, exist to indicate the potential for spread of HIV, first to sex workers and, if the virus accumulates among them, to their clients and on to clients' wives and children. The fact that sporadic testing of a few hundred sex workers who are in custody has not revealed high levels of HIV in most countries should be no excuse for complacency and neglect. As long as these people are not reached with prevention education and specially managed STD services, the national risk will grow. It is important that these aspects be confronted by all concerned parties in a special policy process that seeks a

FIGURE 3.1

Evolution of the Seroprevalence of HIV among Bar Hostesses and Sex Workers between 1987 and 1996 in Djibouti

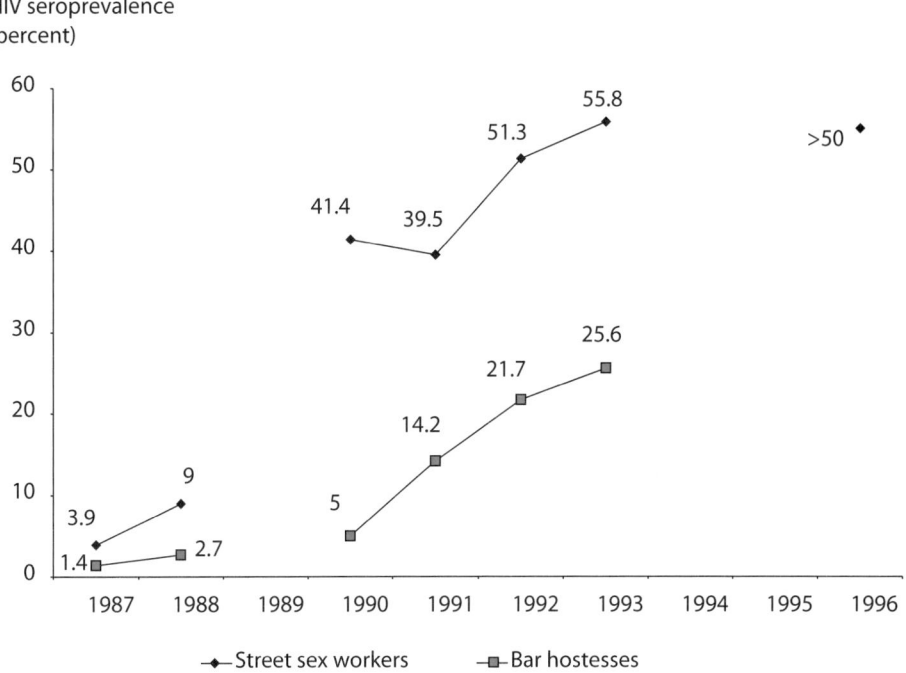

Source: Etchepare 2001.

culturally tolerable level of outreach and service provision for the sake of the public's health.

Men Who Have Sex with Men

As elsewhere, the least acceptable sexual behavior in the region is homosexuality. Strictly forbidden by religious teachings, MSM hide their preferences from family and friends, but homosexual transmission of HIV has been recorded in Algeria, Egypt, Jordan, Kuwait, Lebanon, Morocco, Oman, Qatar, the Republic of Yemen, Syria, and Tunisia, and heightened risk practices are thought to be found in this group (Khan 1995, 1996; Schmitt and Sofer 1992). In Egypt, one of the few countries in which samples of MSM have been repeatedly tested for HIV, prevalence has hovered around 1 percent for the past few years, while MSM represent 32 percent of recently (1997–2001) recorded AIDS cases (USAID/Egypt 2001b) (see box 3.2). While the National AIDS Program recognizes the need for active prevention, the recent publicized arrest of young men who were accused of being involved in homosexual relations has made its efforts more difficult (El Deeb 2001; Fam 2001).

BOX 3.2

Men Who Have Sex with Men, in Egypt

The National AIDS Program (NAP) conducted one small study of 58 MSM in early 1994. This Cairo study was achieved through snowball sampling, producing a strong participation bias toward the well-educated middle class, with 96.5 percent of the men literate, 26 percent university graduates, and 37 percent of professional occupational groups. In this sample, more than 30 percent were married and 44 percent were bisexually active; 20 percent were male sex workers and 67 percent admitted to having more than five male partners concurrently, though only 21 percent ever used condoms, with fewer than 2 percent using them consistently. No organized programs for MSM exist, although socially interconnected groups have been in touch with the NAP. The study's small size and method of sampling indicates a lack of representativeness and points up the importance of further well-conducted social and behavioral research.

Source: El-Sayed and others 1994.

It is maintained, however, that discreet activities can be carried out with MSM for the purposes of HIV prevention. Projects that reach MSM in culturally similar nations do exist, for example, in Morocco (Tawil and others 1999), Pakistan, and Bangladesh (Jenkins, Ahmed, and others 2001), and can provide templates for such projects elsewhere. Following a situational assessment, HIV/AIDS prevention outreach activities have recently been initiated among MSM in Beirut, Lebanon.

Morocco appears to be the first country in the region to have developed HIV prevention programs for male sex workers (Boushaba and Hammich 2000; Boushaba and others 1999); more recently, such a program has been started in Lebanon as well. Not enough is known about the level of commercial male-to-male sex elsewhere in the region.

Vulnerable Groups

For the most part, the behaviors mentioned above are believed to be practiced by a small minority of people who, nevertheless, could spark a more widespread epidemic. The majority of people in all countries are not practicing high-risk behaviors, nor do we expect the majority to become infected with HIV. There are, however, a large number of people in the MENA/EM region, as elsewhere, in a state of vulnerability, which simply means that if certain factors shift in their lives, they will be at risk. Preventing infections in this group is a longer-term investment in overall

health, particularly sexual and reproductive health, and contributes to reducing both adult and infant/early childhood mortality rates as well as the
extraordinary cost of HIV/AIDS to a nation as a whole. In the MENA/EM
region, these groups encompass, among others, migrants (including workers, refugees, and tourists), noninjecting drug users, and youth.

Migrants

It is important to state at the outset that studies indicate that being a migrant per se is not a risk factor for HIV. But the reasons people migrate
and the conditions under which they live during and after migration
often increases vulnerability and can trigger high-risk behavior. Migration for work is largely driven by poverty, unemployment, and a search
for a better livelihood. In the MENA/EM region, the nation with the
largest number of out-migrant workers is Egypt, with an estimated 3
million people, the majority of whom are men, working mostly in the
Gulf countries. Reportedly, between 150,000 and 350,000 people are
screened for HIV yearly before they work abroad. Algeria, the Islamic
Republic of Iran, Jordan, Lebanon, Libya, Morocco, Syria, and Tunisia
also report high levels of out-migration. Exact figures are difficult to obtain, and most experts believe the figures are misleading because the level
of clandestine migration is high everywhere. From the host country perspective, Oman's total population includes 25 percent who are migrants
from South and Southeast Asia. Saudi Arabia hosts 850,000 Filipinos.
AIDS prevention takes on a truly international perspective in such circumstances and requires multisectoral and multinational planning and
cooperation.

Returning migrants have often been among the first men registered
with HIV or AIDS in numerous countries and, after transmitting the infection to their wives, are responsible for many of the first cases of pediatric HIV infection. The associated general pattern appears to consist of
several components. First, where migration is largely to Europe, for example, from the Maghreb, most infections have been associated with injecting drug use. Second, where migration has largely been to the Gulf
countries (or for Lebanon, to West and Central Africa), most infections are
associated with sexual activities, either commercial or otherwise. Third, it
is difficult to prove that returning infected migrants become a core trans-
mitter group. Although some of their wives and newborns may acquire the
virus, the spread from them generally stops there. Changed life circumstances, including learning that one has HIV, appear to effectively diminish risk-taking for many people, and the force of infection does not sustain
an epidemic from this group. There are, however, other concerns because

continuing migration means continuing addition of new infections in home countries, some inevitable transmission to local people, and, more critically, large numbers of uninfected men who return with newly acquired habits, either of drug use or commercial or casual sex.

Well over a million Bangladeshi, Ethiopian, Indian, Philippine, Thai, and Sri Lankan women are contracted as domestic servants, cleaners with various companies and schools, and for other services in the region; a large proportion of these women may be at risk for commercial or coercive sex (Blanchet 2002; Heise, Moore, and Toubia 1996; Khaled 1995). As the women are rarely present for long periods, a quick turnover moves any HIV-infected woman out of these countries rapidly. In Sri Lanka, health authorities estimated in the mid-1990s that up to 40 percent of HIV infections among women involved those who had been working in Gulf states, in particular as domestic workers (WHO/EMRO 2000a). Bangladesh and Pakistan have also documented high rates of HIV among returning migrants from the Gulf regions. Women from the Commonwealth of Independent States (CIS) are also brought in by agencies, and, recently, Bahrain has attempted to crack down on this aspect of the trade (Reuters 2001a). Migrant women are subject to sexual and other abuses around the globe because of their precarious financial and legal circumstances. These issues have been reported repeatedly by the International Office of Migration (IOM), and their mitigation will require excellent international and regional consultation and cooperation.

Short-term or transit migration plays a part in the overall story in some nations. The southern portion of Algeria, having borders with Mauritania, Mali, Niger, and Libya, appears particularly affected (Bouakaz 1998; Bouakaz 2000). At Algeria's Malian and Niger borders, registered migrants rose from 37,054 in 1978 to 61,444 in 1994; in addition, 263,322 people came from Morocco and 851,601 from Libya during these years. These large numbers of people, in addition to the even larger number who are unregistered, often include military men seeking recreation, women seeking work and migrating toward Europe, traders going back and forth, and West and Central Africans in search of work. Because of the commercial market they create, sex workers from elsewhere in Algeria also migrate to the area, which has seen marked rises in reported STD rates and AIDS cases in recent years. Surveillance in the southern border region in 2000 showed that about 1 percent of antenatal women were infected with HIV. The rising local epidemic is understood to create a serious strain on health services in the southern region of Algeria and contribute directly to the risk of HIV spread in the country.

Refugees are an especially vulnerable group of migrants in the MENA/EM region. In the Republic of Yemen, for example, more than 70,000 refugees, mostly from Somalia and Ethiopia, have entered over the past decade (United Nations 2001). Marginalized, poor, and up-rooted, these men and women are vulnerable both to acquiring HIV as well as being deported rapidly if their infections are detected. Despite international conventions, the United Nations High Commissioner for Refugees (UNHCR) must convince any HIV-infected person to be repatriated voluntarily or face incarceration in the Republic of Yemen. A recent assessment (see box 3.3) has shown that the Republic of Yemen has developed little capacity to manage HIV-infected people, whether they are Yemeni or foreign-born.

The reality of refugee vulnerability to HIV is highlighted by the findings of a recent survey in Sudan, which showed that 4.3 percent of a sample of 470 refugees were infected with HIV (Sudan National AIDS Control Program 2001). Little is known about the risks of acquiring HIV among the many Palestinian refugees in the Middle East or the millions of Afghani refugees in the Islamic Republic of Iran and Pakistan. The special problems of HIV prevention and care in conflict situations, as well as postconflict periods, have become increasingly salient and recognized (Hankins and others 2002). Sudan represents an emerging post-conflict situation in which greater freedom and mobility could increase the spread of HIV throughout the country and its neighbors. Recent political circumstances affecting the Middle East and North Africa are likely to worsen this scenario and require considerable attention.

Typically, migrants have less access to health and educational services than residents. AIDS educational campaigns, such as those on World AIDS Day, do not address them, yet they and tourists are easy targets in the common discourse of AIDS as a foreign disease. In Jordan and Egypt, for example, contact between tourists and nationals working in the tourist industry is seen as a situation creating risk of HIV infection. Wherever testing or other studies of local people in the tourist industry have taken place, as in Egypt, there was no evidence of HIV transmission; however, sampling was by convenience and cannot be considered representative. Tunisia has 5 million tourists per year, but local experts recognize that local citizens may be at risk even without contact with tourists.

Tourism among well-off young men in the MENA/EM region may also contribute to the overall risk of HIV spread. It is estimated that Egypt alone receives 1 million Gulf tourists yearly. In a survey of male members of social clubs in Muscat, Oman, in 1995 (n = 245), 13 percent reported extramarital relations over the past 12 months (WHO/EMRO and UNAIDS 2001). One report states that tests of blood donors in the Republic of Yemen showed that HIV was more prevalent among those who had traveled out (1.5 percent) than those who had not (0.05 percent) (U.S. State Department 2001). While adequate in-depth studies have not been undertaken to verify actual patterns, the assumption made most often is that young men (and to a smaller extent, young women) engage in risky sexual behavior when away from home or with foreigners because of the lower risks of discovery. This assumption seems reasonable and, for the past and present time, would help explain the continued low prevalence of HIV in the region as a whole; that is, with the exception of Ethiopia, Thailand, and certain states of India, countries sending workers into the region or countries heavily visited by tourists from the region are themselves low-prevalence countries. This fortunate circumstance cannot be depended on in the future.

Programs to prevent HIV spread among mobile people of all sorts must begin with acknowledging the numerous structural features of vulnerability in each case. These features may include severe poverty in the home country, recruitment by illegitimate brokers, debt bondage, contracts with few safeguards, inadequate legal and other support services, language difficulties, crowded or restrictive living conditions, and, with illegal migration, great reluctance to utilize any services at all. Often migrant workers consider saving money to send home the highest priority, forgoing even the simplest self-care and placing themselves at great risk of abuse from others. Loneliness and the lack of a support network drive many to activities they would not engage in at home, including sex work, pimping, and so forth. Where migrant labor is well organized, these negative features can be minimized, with both sending and receiving countries providing coordinated HIV prevention education and services. Where migration is of the short-term, transit variety, cross-border programs implemented by INGOs and the IOM in the Mekong region of Asia, as well as those supported by the World Bank, UNAIDS, and other partners in West Africa, could serve as models to be examined and adapted for the unique conditions in the MENA/EM region.

Youth

The single greatest factor influencing sexual behavior in all societies is age. Even where social, religious, and cultural values curtail the levels of experimenting with sex before marriage, vulnerability among youth is great. A substantial portion of youth in the region appears to be at risk. In Tunisia, 21 percent of all people with HIV are between 15 and 24 years of age, and 93 percent are single. In Morocco, 63 percent of AIDS cases are among single people, and 40 percent of STDs are recorded among young adults between 15 and 29 years old. The HIV epidemic in Morocco is increasingly reaching young women as often as young men. In Djibouti, among recorded AIDS cases, 3.8 percent are found among those 15 to 19 years old and 43.6 percent among those 20 to 29 years old

(Etchepare 2001; Rodier and others 1990). The sex ratio shows that younger women are more often infected, with 54.3 percent versus 42.7 percent among young men. As these figures from Djibouti reflect infections that occurred 5 to 10 years ago, the early age at which a large proportion of people became infected is striking and disturbing. The tension between maintaining traditional values and modernizing societies through improved educational, health, and communications opportunities is a serious source of social and political conflict. In the MENA/EM region, as elsewhere, religious and other authorities use their influence to counter activities viewed as threatening to the maintenance of traditional forms of social control, particularly those surrounding sexuality, and, even more specifically, female sexuality (Althaus 1997; Anderson 2001; Bourqia 1992; Davis 1992; Ghannam 1997; Ghurayyib 1992; Goodwin 1995; Government of Yemen/UNICEF/World Bank/Radda Barnen 1998; Govindasamy and Malhotra 1994; Guenena and Wassef 1999; Hal 1997; Heikel and others 1999; Heise, Moore, and Toubia 1996; Helmy 1999; Ilkkaracen 2000; International Planned Parenthood Foundation [IPPF] 2001a; Khattab 1996; Khattab, Younis, and Zurayk 1999; Lane 1992; Masterson and Swanson 2000; Mehra and Feldstein 1998; Mernissi 1985, 2000; Obermeyer 2000). Such phenomena as traditional female genital surgery, minimum age at marriage, and related issues have periodically become contentious symbols of this struggle.

Meanwhile, forces of economic globalization and communications proceed apace, with many nations undergoing extremely rapid social and economic changes. The rise in family planning acceptance throughout the region over the past decade or two has significantly reduced fertility almost everywhere (except the Republic of Yemen), and given the demographic momentum, has resulted in a large cohort of youth. In Egypt, Jordan, and Morocco, about one-third of the entire population consists of those between 15 and 29 years of age. Similar proportions are found elsewhere. Coupled with economic forces such as high levels of unemployment among youth nearly everywhere, improved levels of female education, and increasing bride prices in some areas, the average age at marriage has been increasing rapidly in several countries, giving rise to widely acknowledged concerns about HIV vulnerability among the region's youth.

Efforts have been made to conduct knowledge, attitude, and practice (KAP) surveys among youth in Algeria, Djibouti, Egypt, Jordan, Kuwait, Lebanon, Morocco, Oman, Saudi Arabia, Somalia, Syria, Tunisia, the UAE, and elsewhere, but sexual practices were queried in only a few countries (Al Mulla and others 1996; Al-Owaish and others 1999; Essghairi 2000; Family Health International 2001c; Farghaly and Kamal 1991; Faris and Shouman 1994; Gueddána and others 1996; Ministère de la

Santé/PNLS 2001; Ministry of Health in collaboration with UNAIDS and WHO 1999; Petro-Nustas 1999; Reysoo 1999; Saleh and others 2000; Seif El Dawla, Hadi, and Wahab 1998). A recent survey in Sudan has gathered considerable useful behavioral information (Sudan National AIDS Control Program 2002), whereas in Somalia, one survey appears to have not trained interviewers adequately and little useful information on sexual behavior was obtained (WHO/EMRO 2000c). In Djibouti, another study conducted as a stratified sample among 200 young people (100 males, 100 females) at six schools and two out-of-school venues clearly demonstrated the sexual risk-taking of youth, with 71 percent of those between 15 and 19 years old admitting to having had sexual relations (undefined); only 39 percent claimed to have ever used a condom (Ministère de la Santé/PNLS 2001). The data, which are unanalyzed by sex, seem to demonstrate that an increasing proportion of very young people are initiating sexual relations at an early age. Among those currently between 15 and 19 years old, 11 percent admitted to having had their first sexual relations at the age of 13; but among those between 10 and 14 years old, 18 percent stated that they had sex at the age of 13. Discussions about sex and HIV were still considered taboo although, with increasing age, larger numbers of young people had learned about the disease and about condoms.

Less detailed information is available from elsewhere, but a 1994 study in Jordan showed that 7 percent of college students admitted to nonmarital sex, while another national study in 1999 among the general population between ages 15 and 30 showed that 4 percent admitted the same. Among the sexually active, 90 percent mentioned opposite-sex partners only, while 10 percent had partners of either the same sex or of both sexes. Less than half reported ever using condoms. Levels of knowledge about HIV had dropped between surveys (Family Health International 2001c).

In Morocco, qualitative studies seem to show an increasing acceptance of premarital sex among youth, including sex for material exchange, and a certain tolerance of sex work as a means of improving economic status. Simultaneously, young people seem to believe that condoms destroy pleasure and are associated with flagrant misbehavior such as adultery; that admitting to having an STD will lead to punishment, so they prefer to go to pharmacies for treatment because they distrust public facilities; and that AIDS is not yet perceived as a problem for Moroccans (Davis 1992; Farza 2001).

An excellent national study of youth in Egypt did not examine sexual risk-taking but, nonetheless, yielded very useful information (see box 3.3).

Like parents everywhere, MENA/EM parents seem convinced that sexual activity among youth is increasing relative to their own youth. Elsewhere, improved nutrition and health care have been shown to influ-

BOX 3.3

Young People in Egypt

Egypt has the largest population in the Arab world with about 68 million people, and, with a current population growth rate of only 1.72 percent, the demographic momentum has created the largest cohort of youth in Egypt's history. There are at least 13 million young people between the ages of 10 and 19, representing one-fifth of the total population. Educational enrollment has increased at all levels, although marked disparities occur by region. Yet one-third of all 10-year-old girls have never been to school, and 12 percent are married before 19 years old, with an average age at first pregnancy of 17.6 and associated high levels of stillbirths and infant deaths. In some regions, as high as 20 percent of girls are married by age 19. These married adolescents are also often the least educated. Regardless of education, few youths understand the nature of their changing bodies, reproductive functioning, and sexuality.

In 1997, a national survey was conducted of 9,128 adolescents and parents. Results showed that 86 percent of unmarried girls continue to be circumcised, despite a growing conviction that it is not necessary, especially among the more educated. In addition to the gender-biased problems in education and employment that girls face, the study revealed that boys also must handle serious obstacles, including unexpectedly high rates of undernourishment, stunted growth, exposure to violence, and excessive work force participation. On a positive note, many Egyptian youngsters expressed confidence in their future and felt able to discuss a wide variety of topics with their parents, except for sex. Sex education in school is confined to biology, but does not seem to be well executed, given the level of understanding revealed in this survey. Most young people have not learned even basic information from schools, and while they would like to discuss these issues with their families, parents do not feel comfortable giving them this information.

The hotline established in Cairo for AIDS prevention yields evidence that many misconceptions and dangerous gaps in understanding exist. Sexual mores are well understood, and young women know they are expected to preserve their virginity to maintain family honor. Some will be subject to virginity examination at the time of marriage, and therefore practice various ways to avoid discovery. Young men may avoid social approbation through use of sex workers and sex with other males. These realities are known to exist but little progress has been made in addressing them, despite the fact that all concerned recognize they place the coming generation of adult Egyptians at risk of HIV infection.

Source: El-Gawhary 1998; Population Council 1998.

ence the age of sexual maturity, lowering it and creating considerable disjunctive problems with a rising age at socioeconomic maturity. It is likely that this has been occurring in the MENA/EM region as well, although adequate studies have not been conducted to demonstrate this or other factors directly contributing to vulnerability among youth. However, studies in Europe and, more recently, in Uganda and the United States, have shown how improved adolescent education and services can reverse these trends, or, at a minimum, significantly reduce the harm caused by earlier and more frequent premarital sexual activity. Tunisia has taken steps to bring these services to its young; Egypt plans to develop an improved reproductive health program that will incorporate the "life skills"[2] approach. There is clearly a great deal of scope in the region to develop culturally sensitive reproductive health education and services for young people that could affect decisionmaking regarding risky behavior.

Children under specially disadvantaged circumstances must be noted. Refugee children are a case in point, as well as specially marginalized groups such as the caste in the Republic of Yemen known as *Akhdam* (literally meaning "servants"), a historical minority kept at the bottom of society and considered by observers to be at greater risk of acquiring HIV (Republic of Yemen and UNDP 1998; UNICEF 2001b; United Nations 2001). In addition, there are an estimated 200,000 street children in Egypt, and increasingly large numbers working or begging on the streets in the Republic of Yemen (Government of Yemen/UNICEF/World Bank/Radda Barnen 1998), the Islamic Republic of Iran, and elsewhere. Studies suggest that such children are vulnerable to sexual and drug abuse in most cities of the world.

STI/STD Patients

Levels of STIs are generally unknown in the region. Because most infections are asymptomatic in women and many, especially viral infections, are asymptomatic in men, few data exist that would reflect actual prevalence of infections. More commonly, registered patients with disease symptoms (STDs) are reported. Few proper studies of STIs among high-risk groups have been conducted, and where they have, these results usually have not been officially published. Fear and shame continue to characterize STD issues in much of the region.

By law in most countries, STDs are notifiable diseases, but reporting is generally limited, data are confusing, and private practitioners seldom comply. The high level of stigma associated with STDs drives the majority of patients to private practitioners. Furthermore, WHO has encouraged most countries to report using the syndromic method,[3] but the

accuracy of this approach without validation both for treatment and reporting, particularly for women, has been repeatedly questioned (Garg
and others 2001; Hawkes and others 1999; Heikel and others 1999; Ryan
and others 1998). Where assessments have been made of service
providers, preventive counseling and condom promotion and distribution have not been observed. Proper STI surveys are needed in every
country in the region both to document community levels of pathogens
and the main service indicators. Improvement of STD treatment programs is a major investment in HIV prevention.

Anecdotal evidence suggests high levels of STDs in the Republic of
Yemen, but the source of these data has not been found. The Republic
of Yemen has no STD clinics, and women only have access to gynecol-
ogy clinics. The prevalence of syphilis by serology among blood donors
is reported as 2 percent (Global Fund to Fight AIDS, TB, and Malaria
[GFATM] 2002). One study in Jordan found high levels of chlamydia
while another found none. Laboratory issues may be a concern in Jordan
(Family Health International 2001c). In Oman, where health facilities,
including laboratories, are considered to be good, antenatal women are
screened for syphilis, but rates are very low; 2 percent of blood donors
test positive. STIs are reportedly rare in Lebanon, which one study in
the Bekaa Valley seems to confirm (El Nakib 2001; WHO/EMRO
2001b, 2001c). STI/STDs among known high-risk groups, however,
have not been reported. In Syria, syndromic reporting has been introduced in four governorates. These reported 2,342 STD cases for the period of April–June 1999. Other studies have been done but remain unre-
ported (Syrian Arab Republic 2001a, 2001b). In Egypt, some studies
show significant levels of reproductive tract infections (RTIs) among
women, but not necessarily STDs (Khattab and others 1996). More recently, an important study conducted by Family Health International has
shown that 36.5 percent of sex workers (n = 52), 23.8 percent of MSM
(n = 80), 5.3 percent of drug users (n = 152), 8.3 percent of family planning clinic attendees (n = 108), and 4 percent of antenatal clinic attendees (n = 607) had detectable STIs (Family Health International
1998–2000). In Algeria, STD notifications rose in the south between
1990 and 1995 by 22 percent and again in 1996 by 26.7 percent (Bouakaz
2000). In Morocco, increasing numbers of STI cases are reported, but
that may well be the result of increasing coverage of improved STD clinics. It is recognized that at least 50 percent of all patients go to private
practitioners or use self-treatment, and much more work is necessary to
educate the populace about STDs (Heikel and others 1999). Among antenatal women, 1 percent are reported to test positive for syphilis. A
study of 294 secondary students in Djibouti found no syphilis despite the
presence of 46 percent in sex workers (Rodier and others 1993c). In

other words, data are sketchy, do not reflect community levels, and indicate that a considerable proportion of infected people do not seek proper treatment. A summary estimate of STI annual incidence levels for 1999 by region compared with Djibouti shows that reported levels in the MENA region are considerable, even if lower than Djibouti itself and significantly lower than Sub-Saharan Africa (see figure 3.2).

Structural Vulnerability

Structural factors that contribute to risk can be considered to be those that usually affect more than one person and result from the way societal institutions are structured. For example, these factors may include health services and health service policies, the labor market, and education policies, or the structure and functioning of a refugee camp or prison. As in any complex etiology, no one factor is fully determinative, and the conditions in communities with increased vulnerabilty to HIV vary considerably. However, patterns have emerged and regularities are discernable. Where overall social and economic conditions are poor, not only is there a greater chance of HIV spreading, but there also is less capacity to handle both prevention and care.

Measures of larger social and economic factors, such as the Human Development Index, literacy rates by gender, unemployment, expenditures on health and, as a measure of women's health, maternal mortality,

FIGURE 3.2

Estimated Annual Incidence of STIs: Africa, Middle East, and Djibouti

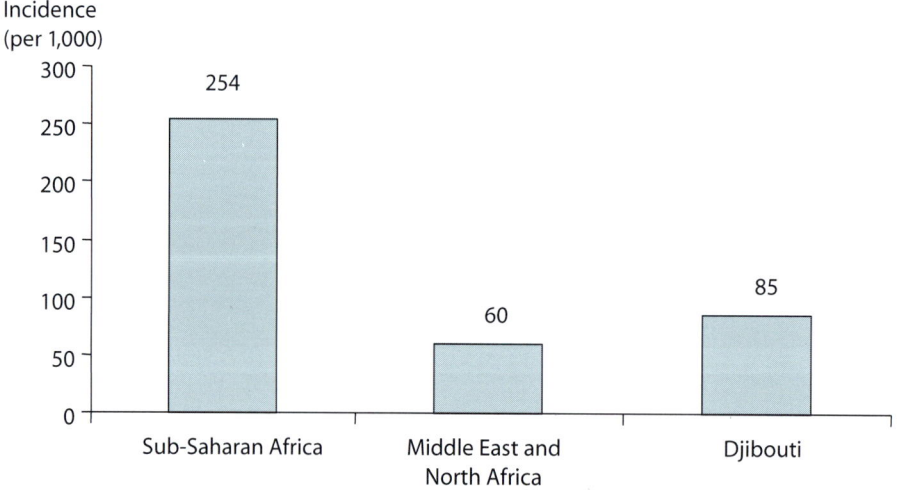

Source: Etchepare 2001.

give an indication of the relative state of development in each country in the region (see table 3.1). The proportion of the population that is urban also is an important indicator of potential vulnerability. Although, ordinarily, all services are better in urban areas, drug use and sex work are both more common in urban than in rural areas.

These indicators, like all such measures, obscure real differences within population segments in a country. For example, although the total proportion of Moroccans living in poverty is estimated variously at between 13 and 16 percent, rural Moroccans are worse off, representing 60 percent of all the poor. This situation drives high levels of internal migration, with increasing numbers of young men and women searching for jobs in urban areas. While the national unemployment rate is 22 percent, the rate is 35.5 percent among youth 15 to 24 years old. Similar disparities are found elsewhere, for example, in Tunisia, with double the rate of unemployment among youth (36 percent for 18- to 19-year-olds, 31.1 percent for 20- to 24-year-olds) compared with overall national figures (16 percent). In Algeria, a general unemployment rate of 30 percent particularly affects young graduates, who may account for 75 percent of total unemployment (World Bank 2002a). With increasing investment in education and stagnating overall economic growth, the levels of unem-

TABLE 3.1

Selected Indicators of Development by Country and Human Development Index

Country	Human Development Index	Male literacy (percent)	Female literacy (percent)	Unemployment	GDP spent on health (percent)	Maternal mortality (percent)	Urban (percent)
Kuwait	35	82	75	—	2.9	5	97
Bahrain	37	89	79	—	5.7	60	92
Qatar	41	79	80	—	2.8	—	90
UAE	43	79	80	—	2.5	26	83
Libya	65	88	63	—	—	220	84
Lebanon	69	95	90	—	5.3	100	86
Saudi Arabia	78	72	50	—	—	130	82
Oman	89	95.5	79	—	—	190	77
Jordan	94	93	79	14	7.9	41	70
Iran, Islamic Rep. of	95	77.5	56.4	12.7	6.0	37	61
Tunisia	102	82	64	16	5.9	70	63
Algeria	109	74	49	30	4.6	160	56
Syrian Arab Rep.	111	87	56	—	—	180	52
Egypt, Arab Rep. of	120	64	39	11.3	1.8	170	45
Morocco	126	62	34	22	3.6	230	52
Yemen, Rep. of	148	63	24	18	1.1	1,400	25
Djibouti	157	73	43	45	7.0	740	82

—Not available.
Source: UNDP 2000; World Bank 2001a, World Bank 2002b.

ployment among college graduates could negatively affect political stability, drug use, and HIV prevalence levels alike.

Rates of literacy are also somewhat misleading with reference to HIV prevention because few of the messages and materials provided by AIDS programs are clear, give explicit information about risk, or even mention the use of condoms for prevention. Most educational efforts are inadequate, and surveys of knowledge among people in the most literate countries reveal large gaps in understanding. For example, in one country, while 71 percent of adolescents aged 16 to 19 reported knowing about HIV/AIDS, only 19 percent knew that condoms are protective. In Jordan, a large survey showed high levels of knowledge about modes of transmission, yet one-third of respondents thought HIV could be acquired from mosquitoes and toilets, and only 29 percent had ever seen a condom. Half of the respondents thought they could see if a person had HIV, an extremely dangerous belief (Family Health International 2001c). A large study in 1999 showed that, while most of the people in Kuwait were aware of the main modes of HIV transmission, a gap existed about modes that did not transmit the disease. This lack of understanding was reflected in their attitudes and practices toward HIV/AIDS patients and a lack of protective behavior change (Al-Owaish and others 1999). In most of the region, media constraints limit discussions. Access to the Internet remains relatively low in much of the MENA/EM region. The lack of access to information is a serious factor increasing vulnerability.

Inequity in resource and income distribution appears to play a major role in fueling HIV epidemics. The exact mechanisms through which this occurs are not clear, but are likely to include differential access to health care, pertinent information, and the power to protect oneself from HIV. Sociological studies have long shown that rising expectations not accompanied by rising opportunities produces fertile ground for socially disruptive forces and movements of many kinds. Stagnant economies and high unemployment among youth lead to increased drug-, violence-, and sex-related risk scenarios. Strong family ties can counter this trend, but where families are weakened by long-term migration, low incomes, or family disruption, youth are unprotected.

Gender bias in educational and employment opportunities specifically places women at an even greater disadvantage. In Uttar Pradesh, India, studies have revealed the close link between domestic violence and the risk a wife has of acquiring an STD from her husband (Martin and others 1999). In Bangladesh, studies suggest that accessing Grameen Bank–type loans plays a role in reducing domestic violence by making women's lives more public (Schuler and others 1996). Women without economic power are less able to protect themselves from the risk of HIV; even more threatening is the fact that most women never perceive that they are at risk of acquiring HIV at all, until it is too late. The highest risk group in any society consists of faithful, uninfected wives married to (unfaithful) HIV-infected husbands. As only a small proportion of men ever reveal their infections (if known) to their wives, these women are thoroughly vulnerable, as are their unborn children. Thus, improving women's economic power can have direct and indirect benefits for HIV prevention.

Inequity in resources takes on new and ominous meanings in the era of AIDS, and governments have an obligation to reduce poverty and provide the means of protection to all their citizens. Long-term investment in reducing the structural factors contributing to vulnerability for HIV infection in the region can only be approached through multisectoral responses. This objective will require a significant effort in planning, through consultative and collaborative processes, appropriate responses that can shore up the gaps that allow HIV to enter social networks and spread.

Notes

1. Others include health workers and multiply exposed patients but, under ordinary conditions, the risk to these groups is easily reduced.

2. Life skills programs have been developed by UNICEF, the United Nations Population Fund (UNFPA), and many other agencies, for both in-school and out-of-school youth. They are locally adapted to the needs of young people, incorporate local values, teach skills, are often peer-led, and view sexual and drug-taking behavior within the larger context of responsible decisionmaking for healthier life styles.

3. Syndromic management and reporting of STDs focuses on symptoms only in an effort to avoid the use of laboratory tests in resource-poor settings.

CHAPTER 4

Assessing the Potential Economic Impact of HIV/AIDS in the MENA/EM Region

The human cost of HIV/AIDS is incalculable, from the pain and guilt surrounding personal and intimate relationships to threatened social and political security at the state level. It is nonetheless instructive to examine those costs that can be calculated, for these too are great and can have a major impact on the future of a nation.

This chapter summarizes the results of an assessment of the potential macroeconomic impacts of HIV/AIDS in selected MENA/EM countries. Where prevalence levels are low, studies of eventual economic implications are useful to demonstrate the costs and losses that will accrue if investments are not made rapidly to avoid the outbreak of an epidemic. As discussed previously, HIV epidemics are sensitive to changing economic and social factors and, in the MENA/EM region, current methods of surveillance are unable to detect changes where they are most likely to take place. Therefore, it is essential to raise awareness for all concerned of the importance of investing now to avoid serious consequences later.

This chapter first summarizes the results of recent research on the socioeconomic determinants of the HIV/AIDS epidemic and extrapolates these results to the case of MENA/EM countries. One of the goals is to assess how current official estimates of prevalence levels compare with those predicted by models on the basis of cross-country data. The chapter then develops and exploits a model of growth to evaluate the potential socioeconomic impacts of the HIV/AIDS epidemic in selected MENA/EM countries. The focus is on output, health expenditures, and poverty. Finally, the chapter assesses the gains from preventive investments made promptly and widely.

Exploratory Analysis of the Socioeconomic Determinants of HIV/AIDS Prevalence Levels

The HIV/AIDS epidemic and economic and social environments are interrelated. On the one hand, social norms and economic incentives and constraints shape individuals' behaviors, which are among the main determinants of the evolution of the epidemic. On the other hand, by affecting the health of individuals, reducing life expectancy, and increasing mortality, HIV/AIDS influences the economy and individuals' behaviors. This discussion of the socioeconomic factors that facilitate the spread of the epidemic is based on the results of two exploratory statistical analyses of cross-country data on HIV/AIDS prevalence levels and indicators such as income per capita, inequality, male and female literacy rates, female labor force participation, the share of tourism in total value added, and migration. Not surprisingly, these macrolevel indicators can only explain part of the international variation in HIV/AIDS prevalence levels. Much of this variation remains unexplained and can be attributed to the heterogeneity of the economic, social, and cultural environments. Nonetheless, the goal of the analysis is not to provide rigorous estimates of the impact that changes in economic growth or income distribution could have on HIV prevalence, which would be a hopeless exercise given our rudimentary knowledge about how the epidemic and the economy interact. Instead, the purpose is simply to identify broad categories of social and economic factors that are likely to influence the diffusion of the epidemic in MENA/EM countries.

The first analysis explores correlations between urban HIV/AIDS prevalence levels and eight socioeconomic indicators (Over 1997). These indicators include a crude measure for the age of the epidemic computed as the time elapsed since the first case was identified, the gross national product per capita, the foreign-born percentage of the population, the percentage of Muslims in the population, the Gini index of inequality,[1] the male-female literacy gap, the urban male-female gender ratio for ages 20 to 39, and the share of military forces in the total urban population. The study uses 1997 data for 17 countries from Sub-Saharan Africa, 15 from Latin America and the Caribbean, 14 from Asia (including India and China), and 4 from the Middle East.

The second analysis, developed for the current study, predicts international variations in HIV/AIDS prevalence levels as a function of income per capita, female participation in the labor force, female literacy, the Gini index of inequality, the share of tourism-related activities in gross domestic product (GDP), and migration. The study uses 1997–99 data for 92 countries, including 27 from Africa, 17 from Asia, 13 from Eastern Europe and Central Asia, 21 from Latin America, 9 from the

Middle East, and 5 from North America and Western and Central Europe. The quantitative results of these studies are summarized in tables A.1 to A.3 in the technical appendix. Below we discuss the main messages. We wish to emphasize that, while the two studies use different data and indicators, both arrive at similar conclusions.

One of the results of the studies is that poverty and income inequality facilitate the diffusion of the HIV/AIDS epidemic, although the exact mechanisms remain unknown. Over's study (1997) shows that HIV prevalence levels increase when income per capita declines and inequality increases. On average, a US$2,000 increase in income per capita is associated with a 4 percentage points' lower level. Similarly, if inequality (as measured by the Gini coefficient) is reduced from 50 to 40 (the difference between Honduras and Malawi), the prevalence level would decrease by 3 percentage points (see figure 4.1). Our analysis also finds a strong correlation between inequality and HIV/AIDS prevalence. The impact of income per capita, however, varies by region.

There are various plausible explanations for the finding that poor countries with an unequal distribution of income are likely to be more vulnerable to the epidemic. The poor have less knowledge about the risks of HIV/AIDS and prevention methods; poor populations may have less freedom to define their choices or behaviors (particularly women); poverty may induce low-income individuals to engage in commercial sex (fueled by migration from rural to urban areas prompted by differentials in expected income); poor men may need to delay marriage and there-

FIGURE 4.1

Poverty, Inequality, and HIV/AIDS Prevalence

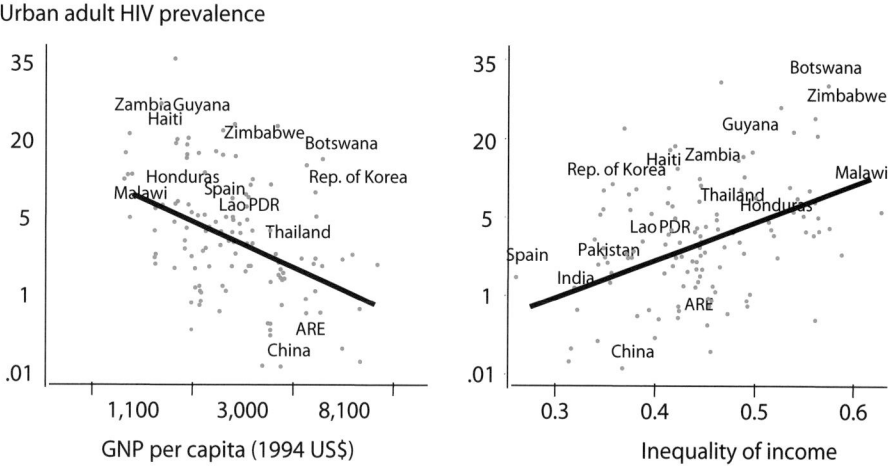

Note: ARE, Arab Republic of Egypt.
Source: Over 1997.

fore delay having a stable partner; and among the poor, spouses may need to leave the household frequently to find jobs. Regardless of the mechanisms, however, international evidence suggests that sustainable growth and a more equal distribution of income are factors that contribute to diminishing the spread of HIV. In MENA/EM, 30 percent of the population is living on less than US$2 per day (see table 4.1). Growth remains elusive, and therefore it is unclear that poverty will retreat over the medium term. Hence, unless actions are taken to tackle HIV/AIDS, the conditions to facilitate the diffusion of HIV epidemics in the region are falling into place.

The studies use various indicators to proxy women's rights in society and provide evidence that gender inequalities are associated with higher HIV/AIDS prevalence. Over (1997) finds that indicators such as the share of female population in urban centers and the gap between male and female literacy rates are correlated with HIV/AIDS prevalence levels. Urban centers where men aged 20 to 39 outnumber women have considerably higher levels of HIV/AIDS prevalence. Countries where women are less educated than men also tend to have higher prevalence (see figure 4.2). Our study finds that, other things being equal, countries with a high female illiteracy rate are also likely to have higher HIV/AIDS prevalence levels. The results also suggest that low female participation rates in the labor force (less than 30 percent) are correlated with high HIV/AIDS prevalence. High participation rates (above 40 percent), however, are also associated with higher HIV prevalence. One possible explanation is that, other things being equal, societies with high female participation in the labor force might also have more liberal sexual behavior. The key message from the analysis is that countries where women are not empowered, and therefore have less or no control over

TABLE 4.1

Population Living on Less than US$2 a Day, by Region

Region	Percentage in 1997	Percentage in 1998	Number in 1987 (million)	Number in 1988 (million)
EAP	67.0	48.7	1,052.3	884.9
ECA	3.6	20.7	16.3	98.2
LAC	35.5	31.7	147.6	159.0
MENA	**30.0**	**29.9**	**65.1**	**85.4**
SA	86.3	83.9	911.0	1,094.6
SSA	76.5	78.0	356.6	489.3
Total	61.0	56.1	2,549.0	2,811.5

Note: EAP, East Asian and Pacific region; ECA, Europe and Central Asia region; LAC, Latin America and Caribbean region; MENA, Middle East and North Africa region; SA, South Asia; SSA, Sub-Saharan Africa
Source: World Bank 2001f.

FIGURE 4.2

Gender Inequality and HIV/AIDS Prevalence

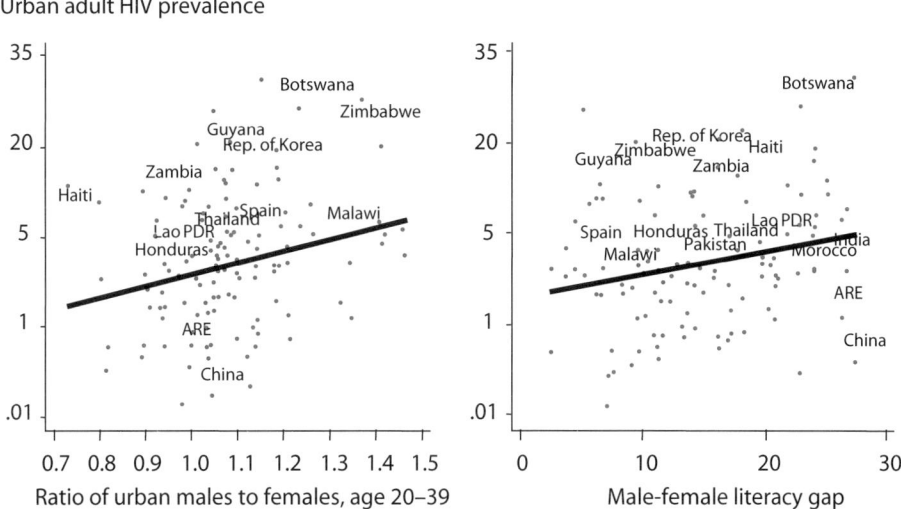

Note: ARE, Arab Republic of Egypt.
Source: Over 1997.

the frequency and type of sexual encounters (in or out of the workplace), provide an ideal environment for the spread of the HIV/AIDS epidemics. These results are backed up by other studies showing that the risk of acquiring an STD for married women is associated with domestic violence (Martin and others 1999). In MENA/EM countries, gender inequalities in terms of access to labor markets and education have been reduced over time. Nonetheless, the gaps are still considerable and this may also contribute to the spread of HIV/AIDS.

Migration and tourism could contribute to the diffusion of HIV, but the evidence from international statistics is not robust. Over's study (1997) on urban HIV prevalence levels finds that countries where 5 percent of the population are immigrants (implying a more important flow of immigrants) can have an HIV/AIDS prevalence level that is 2 percentage points higher than the prevalence of a country with no immigration. However, migration per se is not the risk factor. Risks are determined by the recruitment, labor, and living conditions for migrants in host countries and, importantly, the differential in HIV prevalence levels between source and destination communities. Nonetheless, as the density of flow increases, the probability increases of finding migrants who become part of high-risk groups.

Migration and tourism can also contribute to fueling the epidemic by creating interaction channels with high-risk population groups in other countries affected by HIV/AIDS. However, despite the intuitive sound-ness of these arguments, when looking at the role of tourism and migra-tion, our study does not find statistically significant correlations with HIV/AIDS prevalence levels. One explanation is that in countries that are more exposed to the risk of increased tourism (Thailand), public in-terventions not accounted for in the model have been put into place to reduce HIV prevalence levels. Furthermore, differences in the HIV prevalence in source and destination countries will affect the outcome. Another explanation is that the potential negative effects of increased tourism on HIV prevalence are neutralized by the positive effects on higher economic growth. In MENA/EM countries, both migration and tourism are essential parts of the economy. As liberalization takes place and restrictions on trade and capital flows are reduced, migration and tourism are expected to increase, thus bringing economic benefits. Col-lective risk will be enhanced, though, where part of the tourism is related to commercial sex or drug use, or when migrants access or act as sex workers.

When the model developed for this study is applied to MENA/EM countries, it predicts prevalence rates that are higher than current offi-cial estimates.[2] Given current levels of output per capita, participation of women in the labor force, the level of income inequality, and rates of fe-male illiteracy, HIV prevalence levels in MENA/EM countries could be between 0.2 and 1 percentage point higher than current estimates (see figure 4.3). The predicted prevalence levels are sensitive to model spec-ification but, in all cases, they are higher than those currently reported. Differences could be explained by the absence of appropriate surveil-lance systems.

Potential Socioeconomic Consequences of the HIV/AIDS Epidemic

The more visible impact of HIV/AIDS is on health and life expectancy. It is estimated that in countries with relatively high prevalence levels (above 5 percent), life expectancy has been reduced to the levels observed 10 years ago (World Bank 2000e). Worldwide, while the share of deaths from infectious diseases is expected to decrease from 30 percent today to 14 percent in 2020, the share of these deaths from AIDS could increase during the same period from 2 percent today to 14 percent (Murray and Lopez 1996). AIDS is, of course, not the only health problem. Malnu-trition and childhood-related diseases are currently responsible for more than 1.8 million deaths per year. TB kills 2 million people per year and malaria close to 800,000. It is expected that the number of deaths caused

FIGURE 4.3

Potential Underestimation of Current HIV/AIDS Prevalence in Selected MENA/EM Countries

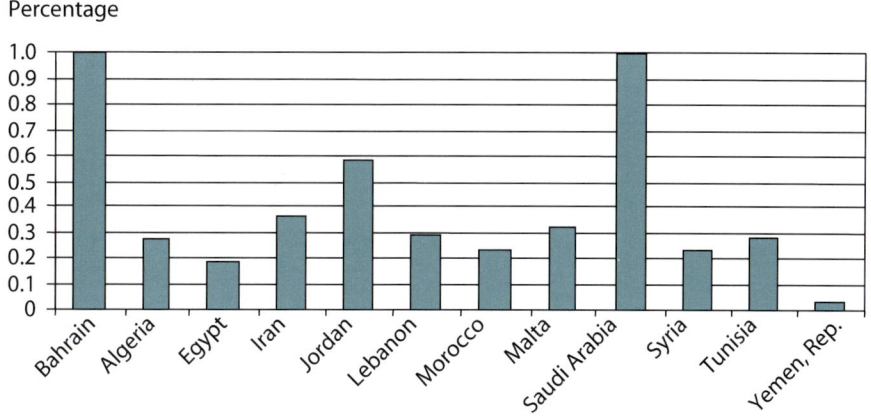

Source: Authors' calculations.

by tobacco will increase from 3 million today to 8.4 million in 2020 (Murray and Lopez 1996). The particularity of HIV/AIDS is that the health impacts are likely to concentrate on young adults in their most productive ages. Thus, AIDS could become the second major cause of death among adults of working age in the world, posing a serious economic threat. Below, we discuss potential implications as they relate to MENA/EM countries.

Economic impacts through the loss of human capital. One channel through which HIV/AIDS affects the economy is by disrupting the human capital accumulation process. Indeed, the human capital of a country is given by the size and quality of its labor force. HIV/AIDS is likely to affect both. First, there are effects in the size and productivity of the current labor force because of higher mortality and morbidity. Premature deaths represent not only losses in a productive factor, but also losses of the knowledge and experience embedded in it. Higher morbidity can also reduce labor productivity, for instance, through high labor turnover (see figure 4.4), higher health insurance expenditures, and the need to put in place preventive measures.[3] Second, HIV/AIDS can affect the accumulation of future human capital. Indeed, premature deaths tend to increase the number of orphans who are less likely to fully develop their physical and intellectual capacities.[4] More important, in the absence of appropriate social protection systems, the income shock associated with the death of a household member, particularly if he or she is the main provider of income, can reduce investment in health, education, and nutrition for children (see Bell, Devarajan, and Gersbach 2003). Shorter life ex-

FIGURE 4.4

HIV/AIDS Prevalence and Worker Turnover

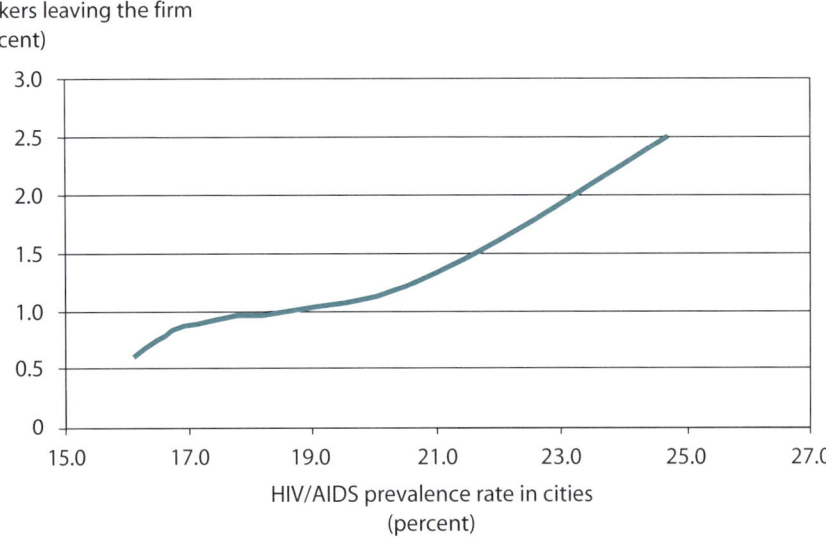

Source: Biggs and Shah 1996.

pectancies resulting from higher mortality also reduce incentives to invest in education and health.

Economic impacts through lower efficiency. The need to finance additional health expenditures and reallocate resources toward curative and preventive measures may also reduce economic efficiency. The impact of the epidemics on the health system is likely to vary widely from one country to another, depending on the type of technologies and services provided to HIV/AIDS patients. In general, however, the epidemic will bring higher demand for health services, increased health care costs, and therefore higher expenditures. The macroeconomic consequences will depend, in part, on how additional expenditures are financed. In the case of public expenditures, governments will have to choose between increasing taxes, issuing debt, or simply reducing other types of expenditures (consumption or investment). For instance, higher expenditures in HIV/AIDS curative interventions could crowd out other health or education expenditures (see figure 4.5). Higher private expenditures could also be financed either by reducing savings[5] or substituting consumption. If lower savings dominate, then new investments and growth would be compromised. In all cases, necessary adjustments to finance additional health expenditures are likely to decrease welfare. Efficiency losses may also result as private and public resources used to supply HIV/AIDS-related services are reallocated away from other more productive uses.

FIGURE 4.5

Annual Cost of Treating an AIDS Patient versus Annual Cost of Primary Education

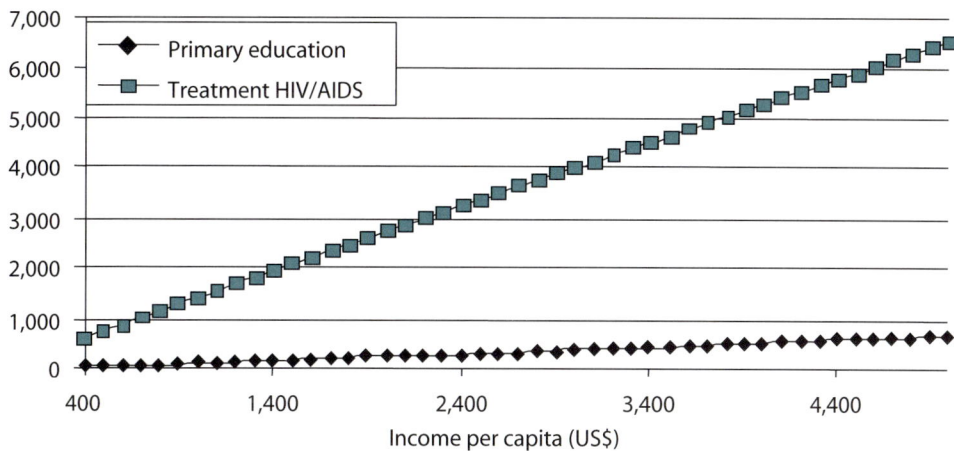

Cost per person per year (US$)

Note: HIV/AIDS expenditures as a function of income per capita in US$ (Y) are given by:

$$\ln E_{aids} = 0.63931 + 0.95 \ln Y$$

Primary education expenditures as a function of income per capita in US$ (Y) are given by:

$$\ln E_{edu} = -3.3554 + 1.1589 \ln Y$$

Source: Cyrillo, Paulani, and Aguirre 2001; Floyd and Gilks 2001; World Bank 2002b.

Empirical studies measuring the economic impact of AIDS find contradictory evidence. Some studies find no correlation between HIV/AIDS prevalence levels and economic growth (Bloom and Mahal 1995). Other researchers (Bonnel 2000) find that growth rates in Africa's most affected countries could have been higher by 1 percentage point in the absence of HIV/AIDS. Most macroeconomic simulation models, however, predict that reductions in economic growth in affected countries could average 0.5 percentage point per year (Ainsworth and Over 1994). Recently it has been argued that by ignoring the impact of the epidemic on the accumulation of future human capital, most studies are underestimating the long-term economic costs (see Bell, Devarajan, and Gersbach 2003). Regardless, short-term economic impacts will depend on several factors, including the severity of the epidemic, the degree to which HIV/AIDS expenditures are financed from savings, the distribution of HIV/AIDS infections by workers' productivity level, the time lost from work by the person with AIDS, and the efficiency of labor markets. In general, *short-term macroeconomic* impacts would be lower in countries with high unemployment rates. This is the case in MENA/EM countries where today's unemployment rates are high, with official rates attaining

21 percent in Algeria and more than 30 percent in Djibouti and the Republic of Yemen. In these cases, the slowdown in the growth rate of the labor force could be translated into a reduction in the unemployment rate and not GDP. Nonetheless, it is important to acknowledge that whether employed or not, a young adult is a potentially productive resource. Thus, the death of an unemployed person is still a loss of human capital.

To evaluate the economic cost of HIV/AIDS in MENA/EM countries, we use a model of growth that includes an HIV/AIDS diffusion component that formalizes transmission through two channels: sexual intercourse and the exchange of infected needles among IDUs. The model is necessarily a simplification of the complex mechanisms through which the economy and the HIV/AIDS epidemic interact.[6] Nonetheless, it is able to capture the impact of the epidemic on (a) the size of the labor force, (b) labor productivity growth, (c) health expenditures, and (d) the savings rate of the economy. A schematic representation of the model is shown in figure 4.6. A more formal presentation of the model is provided in the technical appendix.

The model was calibrated to nine MENA/EM countries (Algeria, Djibouti, Egypt, the Islamic Republic of Iran, Jordan, Lebanon, Morocco, the Republic of Yemen, and Tunisia) on the basis of recent demographic and economic data and projections used in the World Bank Country Assistance Strategies (World Bank 1997a, 1997b, 1999b, 1999c, 2000c, 2001b, 2001c, 2001d; World Bank Group 2001) and the Algeria Social Expenditures Review (World Bank 2002a).[7] The period of analysis is 2000–25. The model is not used for prediction purposes, but rather to explore the likelihood of a large number of plausible futures and associated economic costs. Hence, for each of the countries, we simulate the dynamics of the economy for 100 combinations of the model parameters that determine the diffusion of the epidemic and its economic impacts: the shares of high risk populations (IDUs and sex workers); the HIV/AIDS prevalence rates among these groups; the frequency and heterogeneity of sexual interactions; the prevalence of STDs, the prevalence of condom use and needle sharing; and the distribution of AIDS-related deaths among unemployed, skilled, and unskilled workers, as well as the reduction in total factor productivity resulting from an increase in the HIV/AIDS prevalence rate (see the technical appendix for a description of the methods used to calibrate the model).

As an illustration, figure 4.7 presents two HIV/AIDS diffusion profiles for a typical MENA/EM country. The profiles depend on the prevalence of condom use, the level of access to safe needles among IDUs, the presence of STDs, and the intensity and heterogeneity of sexual behaviors. Clearly, there are high levels of uncertainty in terms of how the epidemic is likely to diffuse. This level of uncertainty is captured in the case

FIGURE 4.6

A Model of Growth to Evaluate the Macroeconomic Impacts of HIV/AIDS

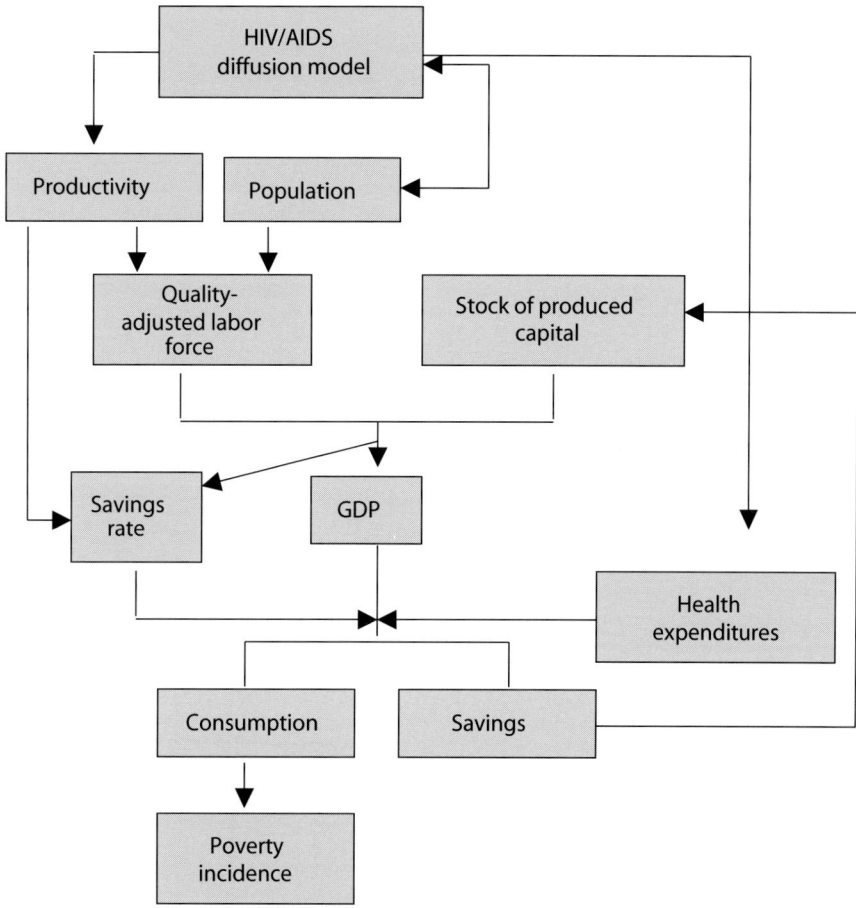

Source: Authors' design.

of Jordan in figure 4.8. Each bar in the figure is associated with a given prevalence rate. The height of the bar gives the number of scenarios that generate that particular prevalence rate. We observe that the prevalence rate could range anywhere from 0 to more than 20 percent. However, more likely, the prevalence rate in 2015 would be below 5 percent. As we will see, the challenge for policymakers is to reduce this level of uncertainty and to insure against it.

We need to make two important assumptions to assess the impact on the economy of the various paths that the epidemic can take. First, in terms of the distribution of HIV infections among unemployed, skilled, and unskilled workers, second regarding the link between HIV preva-

FIGURE 4.7

Illustration of Diffusion Profiles for the HIV/AIDS Epidemic in MENA/EM Countries

Profile 1: Low Risk

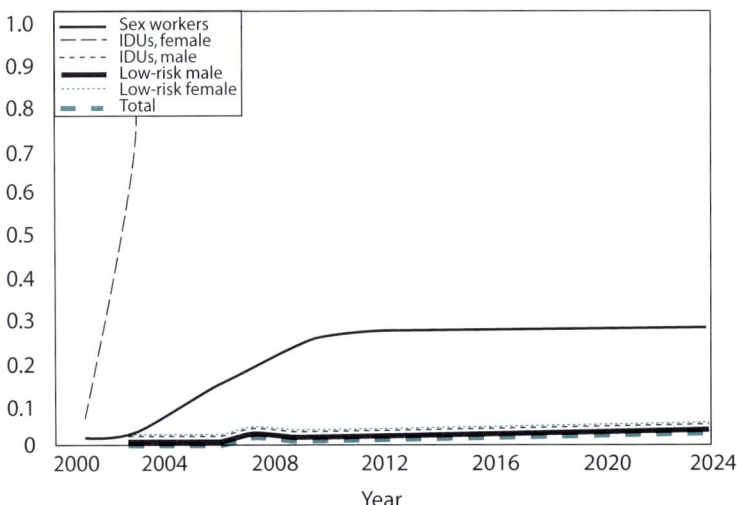

Profile 2: High Risk

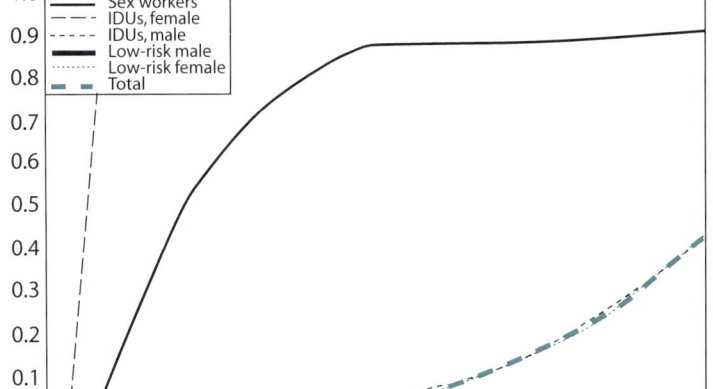

Note: We assume that only high-risk individuals are infected initially. In Profile 1, we consider a 50 percent prevalence of condom use, only a 10 percent probability of sharing needles among IDUs, 1 percent STD prevalence, low sexual activity and low heterogeneity (as reflected by the parameters in table A.4 in the technical appendix). In this case, the epidemic is mostly confined to high-risk population groups, particularly IDUs, where within a few months all the population is infected. In Profile 2, condom use drops to 10 percent, the STD prevalence increases to 5 percent, and the parameters defining sexual behaviors are multiplied by 1.5. Now the epidemic spreads to the general population and attains alarming levels among sex workers.
Source: HIV/AIDS diffusion model.

FIGURE 4.8

Jordan: Plausible Predictions for HIV/AIDS Prevalence

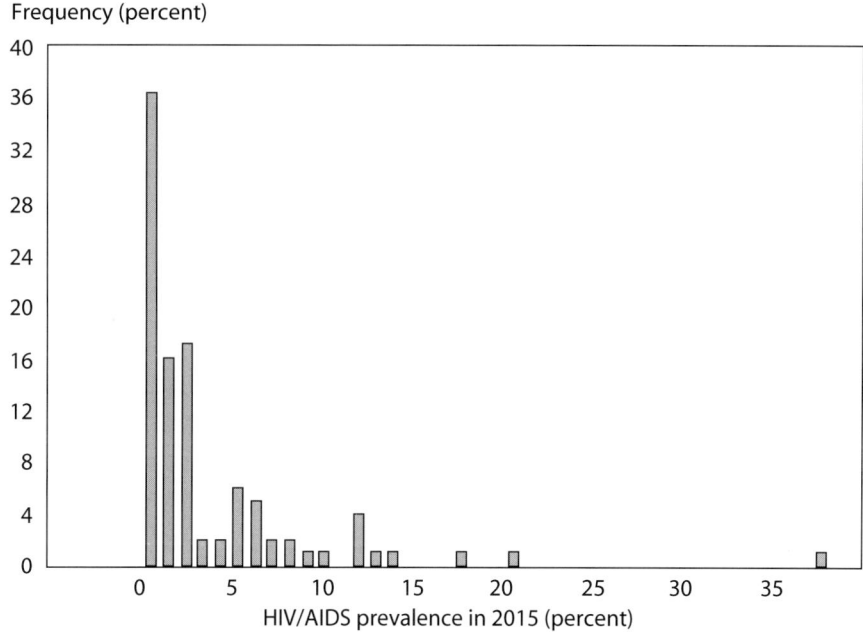

Note: Each bar is associated with a given HIV/AIDS prevalence rate. The height of the bar gives the number of scenarios that generate the given prevalence rate.
Source: Authors' calculations.

lence and total factor productivity growth. There are few data to cali-brate these parameters. Hence, as in the case of the parameters deter-mining diffusion scenarios, we consider a large number of combina-tions.[8] For each combination of a diffusion profile and an impact scenario, we compute five output variables: the present value[9] of total GDP produced between 2002 and 2025, the average growth rate of GDP for that period, the size of the population in 2025, and the HIV/AIDS prevalence level and total share of AIDS-related health ex-penditures in GDP in 2015. Given the lack of epidemiological data, there is a wide range of variation for the outcome variables. Descriptive statistics for these variables are presented in table A.7 in the technical ap-pendix. Here we discuss the main messages.

In terms of the HIV/AIDS prevalence rate, we find several scenarios where it fluctuates around 4 percent by year 2015 (see technical appendix figures A.1–A.5). The fact that prevalence rates are similar across coun-tries reflects little variation in epidemiological initial conditions. The ex-ception is Djibouti, where the prevalence rate is already at 3 percent and could reach 15 percent by 2015 (see table 4.2). In general, once the

TABLE 4.2

Economic Impacts of the HIV/AIDS Epidemic

(average across agencies)

	Present value losses 2000–25 (percent GDP)	Average reduction in GDP growth (percent)	Population change in 2025 (percent)	HIV prevalence in 2015 (percent)[a]
Algeria	41.22	−0.40	−4.07	4.46
Djibouti	150.77	−1.34	−16.68	15.88
Egypt, Arab Rep. of	51.33	−0.42	−3.84	4.23
Iran, Islamic Rep. of	38.65	−0.42	−3.85	4.18
Jordan	33.56	−0.35	−3.16	3.69
Lebanon	30.03	−0.45	−4.44	4.63
Morocco	39.48	−0.42	−3.97	4.27
Tunisia	54.04	−0.44	−4.21	4.43
Bahrain	35.58	−0.38	−3.92	4.20
Kuwait	35.70	−0.36	−3.78	4.11
Oman	35.56	−0.35	−3.63	4.04
Qatar	33.19	−0.38	−4.00	4.27
Saudi Arabia	35.84	−0.31	−3.12	3.72
UAE	25.57	−0.32	−3.40	3.91

a. HIV/AIDS are not projections but simple averages across scenarios.
Source: Authors' calculations.

HIV/AIDS epidemic reaches 4 percent, its development becomes exponential. Hence, across scenarios, the accumulated economic costs for the period 2000–25 could approximate 30 to 50 percent of GDP (greater than 150 percent in the case of Djibouti). In all countries it is possible to find scenarios, although rare, where accumulated costs surpass current GDP. GDP losses reflect the slowdown in the GDP growth rate, which in most countries could approximate 0.4 percentage point per year (this is in line with the value found by other studies). Hence, the impacts on economic growth can be substantial, even if most of the countries face high unemployment rates. Costs could be even higher than those reported here, if we had accounted for the impact of the epidemic on the accumulation of future human capital.

Because the epidemic is still in its early stages, projected demographic impacts seem relatively small. For instance, in the case of Jordan and the Republic of Yemen, the size of the labor force would be reduced by 3 percent in 2025. In Algeria, the Islamic Republic of Iran, and Morocco, this number would be closer to 4 percent. This is equivalent to a reduction in the average population growth rate of 0.1 to 0.3 percentage point per year.[10] Since the slowdown of the economies is also accompanied by a reduction in population growth rates, the overall impact in the growth rate of GDP per capita is less severe. In some extreme cases, this growth rate could even increase as a result of the epidemic. This would happen if the negative impact of HIV/AIDS on population growth rates was considerably higher than its impact on economic growth. Thus, caution is needed when using GDP per capita as an indicator of the economic impacts of the HIV/AIDS epidemic.[11]

Impacts on Health Expenditures

Given a diffusion profile, the impact of the epidemic on health expenditures will depend on the average cost of treating an AIDS patient and the share of the population of patients who have access to treatment. Little information is available about these two factors in MENA/EM countries, and, therefore, the calculation of potential changes in health expenditures is based on estimates from the literature. In terms of the average cost of treatment, estimates from cross-country studies suggest a range of two to three times GDP per capita, excluding the cost of antiretroviral drug (Cyrillo, Paulani, and Aguirre 2001; Floyd and Gilks 2001). In this analysis, we work under the conservative assumptions that the average yearly cost of treating an HIV/AIDS patient is equal to US$1,400 in a country with a GDP per capita of US$1,000, and that it increases by 0.95 percent for each 1 percent increase in GDP per capita. Access to treatment, however, varies widely across countries. The results summarized in this section are based on the assumption that 30 percent of those affected by AIDS would obtain treatment.

The simulations confirm that HIV/AIDS could have a significant impact on health expenditures. Across countries, these expenditures could increase by 1.5 percent of GDP, even if only one-third of the patients have access to health services (see figure 4.9). In the case of Djibouti, health expenditures could attain 6.4 percent of GDP. Notice that these numbers are averages across simulations. However, it is possible that even in countries where current prevalence levels are below 1 percent, health expenditures could increase by up to 5 percent of GDP (see the technical appendix, table A.7).

These results are consistent with estimates from the literature that suggest that the major economic consequences of the epidemic would be felt within the health system. For instance, it has been found in the case of India (Ellis, Alam, and Gupta 1997) that a severe AIDS epidemic would increase government health care expenditures by US$2 billion per year. Thus, according to the study, by 2010 health expenditures in India would be 60 percent higher than without HIV/AIDS.

While the analysis developed in this section is highly simplified, it illustrates that the HIV/AIDS epidemic, if uncontrolled, could force important budgetary reallocations. As discussed previously, by taking re-

FIGURE 4.9

HIV/AIDS-Related Average Health Expenditures in 2015
(percentage of GDP)

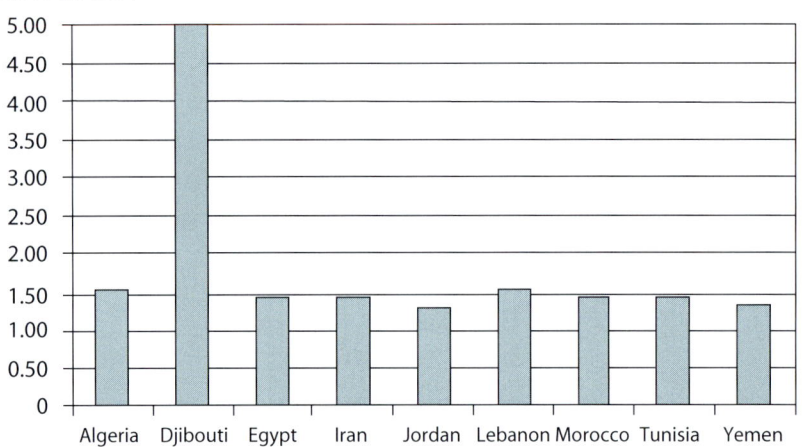

AIDS-related health
exp. in 2015 (% GDP)

Source: Authors' calculations.

sources away from more productive economic activities, such as children's education, these reallocations can reduce aggregate economic efficiency and put additional pressures on long-term economic growth.

Implications for Poverty Reduction

The epidemic will have direct and indirect implications for poverty reduction. First, the epidemic, which is likely to affect disproportionately more low-income individuals, will increase vulnerability and poverty. Second, by slowing down economic growth it will reduce the opportunities that the poor have to escape poverty. We discuss each of these effects in turn.

For the poor and many households with consumption levels just above the poverty line, the main or only source of revenue is their labor. While the nonpoor can hedge their losses in wage income resulting from AIDS with other assets, coping mechanisms for the poor and vulnerable are more limited and usually involve changes in consumption patterns (reducing education, food, and health expenditures) or sending children to work. These mechanisms result in human capital loss as a result of high child malnutrition or lower school enrollment rates, among others. Although informal coping mechanisms to manage risks are diverse in MENA/EM countries—ranging from family support and kinship ties to religious charitable organizations—research has shown that they are usually insufficient to hedge against adverse shocks (World Bank 2001g). Studies show that reductions in consumption in low-income households following the death of an adult household member would reduce food expenditures by 32 percent and food consumption by 15 percent (Over and others 2001). This occurs not only as household income is lost and funeral expenditures need to be financed (on average, households spend 50 percent more, or US$800 to US$900, on funerals than they do on medical care), but also because households that experience a death cut back on the number of hours they work for wages (Biggs and Shah 1996). Hence, HIV/AIDS can be the shock that drives many vulnerable households into poverty. In most MENA/EM countries, the poor already face problems of access to health services. As health systems become financially constrained, these problems can be exacerbated. At the same time, the poor are more exposed to infectious diseases, and, given complications from undernutrition, are more vulnerable to the deterioration of their immune system.

Even among poor households that are not directly affected by the epidemic, the associated slowdown in economic growth will reduce their opportunities to escape out of poverty. Indeed, the evolution of the poverty prevalence of a country is determined by the growth rate of average income and the change in income distribution. Research has shown that income distribution remains relatively unchanged over 10-year periods. Therefore, it is mainly economic growth that determines how many people are lifted out of poverty. In general, a 1 percent increase in per capita income can be associated with a 1 percent to 2 percent reduction in poverty prevalence (Dollar and Kraay 2001). As an illustration, if the growth rate of GDP per capita is reduced by 0.5 percent to 1 percent as a result of HIV/AIDS, the number of people who fail to escape poverty could reach 20 million by 2010. In 1998, close to 30 percent of people in MENA/EM countries (85 million) were living on less than US$2 per day. With an average growth rate of 3 percent per year, by 2010, poverty prevalence could be reduced to somewhere between 22 percent and 16 percent (depending on how sensitive the poverty prevalence is to the growth rate of income per capita), and the number of poor could fall to somewhere between 79 million and 58 million. Because of HIV/AIDS, however, poverty prevalence would be higher in 2010 as the average growth rate of GDP per capita falls by 0.2 percentage point to 1 percentage point (depending on the severity of the epidemic and its impact on labor productivity). The number of people who would have failed to escape poverty could then range between 8 million and 30 million, depending on how sensitive poverty prevalence is to economic growth (see figure 4.10).[12]

Policy Implications

The HIV/AIDS epidemic in MENA/EM presents a typical problem of decisionmaking under conditions of high uncertainty. Prevalence levels could remain at low levels, but there is also a risk that the epidemic could develop through profiles similar to the ones discussed in the previous section, and the human and economic costs could be considerable. We show that waiting to intervene can be costly. Societies are better off if they invest today in interventions to reduce and mitigate the risk of an HIV/AIDS epidemic.

Governments, whose mandate is to ensure the well-being of the population, have the responsibility to develop and finance the implementation of policies to confront HIV/AIDS. Indeed, individuals alone could not devise appropriate mechanisms to contain the epidemic. First, individuals do not take into account the social costs of the risks they take, or the social benefits of the preventive measures they adopt. In the absence of government intervention, we would observe an excess of risky behavior and too little prevention from a social point of view. Second, individuals suffer from information problems. Individuals may not have enough information about the risks of HIV and may lack knowledge and skills related to preventive behaviors. Finally, formal and informal institutions (culture or religious values) may constrain individuals' actions in ways that render them, and society, more vulnerable to HIV/AIDS. The role

FIGURE 4.10

Number of People in the MENA/EM Region Who Would Remain below the Poverty Line as a Consequence of HIV

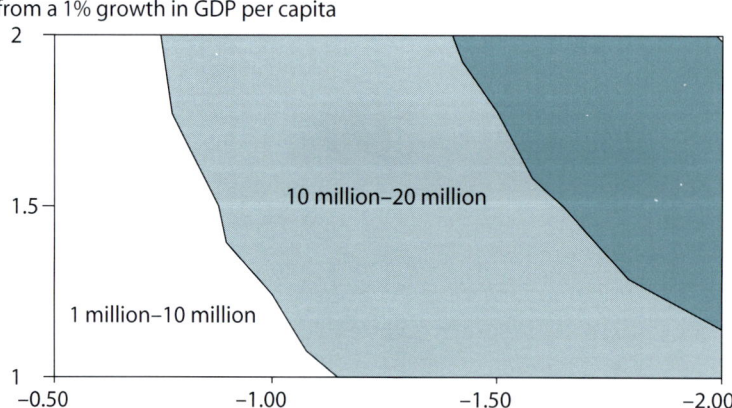

Source: Authors' calculations.

of governments is therefore critical in providing information, subsidizing interventions to reduce risky behaviors, providing care and support for people living with HIV and AIDS (PLWHA), reducing stigma and discrimination, as well as creating the enabling environment.

Governments can only intervene, however, if there are cost-effective interventions at their disposal (Kremer, 1996a, 1996b). Fortunately, international experience has demonstrated that there are cost-effective interventions to tackle HIV/AIDS. Recent studies and collective experience from countries show that interventions can be highly cost-effective when focused on reducing risks (through information and preventive behaviors and services) in those population groups most likely to contract and spread HIV (Jenkins, Rahman, and others 2001; Kahn 1996). Interventions such as reproductive health and HIV/AIDS education in schools, provision of basic prevention and care packages for highly vulnerable groups (including STD treatment), and harm reduction for IDUs have also proved to be cost-effective. To implement these interventions, several instruments are available, including direct provision of services, subsidies, taxes, and regulatory power. In general, early interventions bring higher benefits and lower costs.

In the case of MENA/EM countries, we simulate the impact of increasing condom use by 30 percent and expanding access to safe needles for IDUs by 20 percent (see the technical appendix, tables A.8 and A.9, for a description of the methods used in the simulation and the costs of the interventions). The policy is assumed to be implemented immediately and is applied to each of the 100 scenarios discussed in the previous sections. The results show that these two interventions can considerably reduce GDP losses for the period 2002–25 (see figure 4.11). Across countries, savings (net of the costs of the interventions) could surpass 15 percent of today's GDP (see also tables A.10 and A.11 in the technical appendix). On average, this translates into an increase of 0.3 percentage point in the yearly GDP growth rate. We have also simulated implementing these two interventions with a delay of five years. Not surprisingly, waiting to intervene can cost countries an average of 8 percent of today's GDP (5.6 percent in the case of Djibouti).

In the previous simulations, we have applied the same policy to all countries in all scenarios and this is likely to underestimate net benefits. Indeed, the total amount of resources that societies ought to invest to fight HIV/AIDS and their allocation across alternative interventions depends on countries' characteristics. For instance, in the case of the Republic of Yemen, the simulated intervention may be too costly. In general, the costs and effectiveness of the different interventions are given by factors such as the level of development of the epidemic, social and economic constraints on safe behavior, underlying patterns of

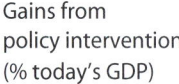

FIGURE 4.11

Benefits from Expanding Access to Condoms and Safe Needles for IDUs and Costs of Delaying Action

Gains from
policy intervention
(% today's GDP)

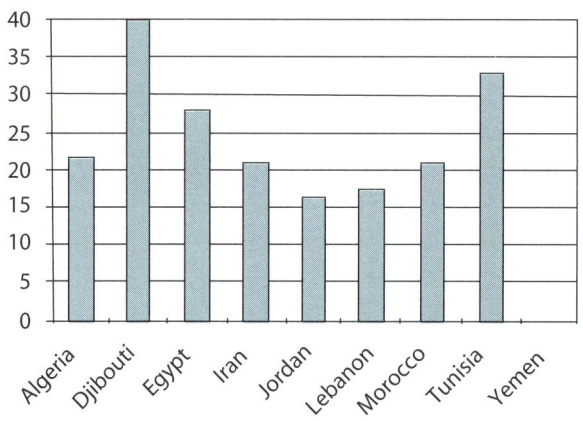

Losses from
5 years' delay
(% GDP)

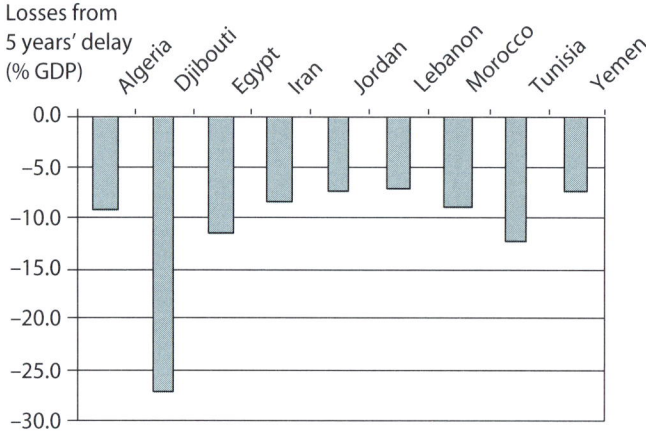

Source: Authors' calculations.

sexual and drug-injecting behavior, local costs, and implementation capacity.

It is not a trivial exercise to decide how many resources to allocate to HIV/AIDS-related interventions and, as important, how to finance this allocation. Indeed, in most countries in the region, health budgets are already under strain. Governments face competing demands not only in the health sector, but also in education and social protection. At the same time, given the potential costs of the epidemic, societies cannot afford to ignore the issue. Our recommendation is to start with small investments to improve current surveillance systems and build knowledge about the current epidemiological situation, for instance, by conducting surveys of zero prevalence and sexual behaviors. Foreign financing is usually available for this type of intervention. Once there is a better understanding of the epidemiological situation (the level of uncertainty discussed in the previous section has been reduced), governments, in coordination with civil society and communities, can initiate the development of a national strategy to prevent a major outbreak. Several methodologies to select and allocate resources across interventions are now available to guide this work (Kaplan and Pollack 1998). Programs that are implemented should be carefully monitored to evaluate costs and impacts, thus allowing adjustments and corrections when necessary. The next chapter discusses some of the interventions that could be considered.

The main messages from this chapter can be summarized as follows: (a) the risk of an increase in the HIV/AIDS prevalence level in MENA/EM countries is real; (b) the expected costs over the next 25 years could be considerable—on the order of 30 percent of current GDP even under conservative assumptions; (c) actions can be implemented to prevent the spread of the epidemic, and the costs of these actions, would be more than compensated by the savings they generate; and (d) the time to act is today, when prevalence levels are still low. Over the short run, governments could consider:

- Investing resources to improve the understanding of the epidemiological situation, as well as key factors that determine its dynamics, such as sexual behaviors.

- Funding interventions that target vulnerable groups or those most likely to be infected with and spread HIV.

- Financing preventive interventions not only in the health sector but also across sectors, such as in education.

Notes

1. The index can have values between 0 and 100. A value of 0 means that the distribution of income is completely equitable: each individual receives an equal share of the national income. A value of 100 implies a completely unequal distribution where one individual receives all the national income. At the international level, the Gini coefficient varies between 21.7 (Belarus) and 59.6 (Guatemala).

2. Predicted rates are based on the most recent WHO/UNAIDS estimates.

3. In countries with high unemployment rates, these costs are likely to be lower (Biggs and Shah 1996).

4. Research has shown that beyond the psychological impacts, among low-income populations, the death of one parent is associated with a deterioration of nutritional status and lower school enrollment rates (Ainsworth and Koda 1993).

5. Private savings can also be reduced if HIV/AIDS increases discount rates, thus favoring present consumption (see the technical appendix).

6. For applications of similar models to the analysis of macroeconomic impacts in other countries, see Bollinger, Stover, and Nalo 1999; Cuddington 1993; Haacker 2001; Hancock and others 1996; Kambou, Devarajan, and Over 1992; Leighton 1993, 1996; Lewis 2000; MacFarlan and Sgherri 2001; Nalo and Aoko 1994; Over 1998; Quattek 2000; Robalino, Voetberg, and Picaso 2002.

7. The model was also used to estimate reductions in GDP growth in selected Gulf countries (Bahrain, Kuwait, Oman, Qatar, Saudi Arabia, and the UAE). No other analyses were conducted in the case of these countries, given data constraints.

8. We allow for alternative distributions of new infections: the share of total deaths occurring among skilled workers is allowed to vary between 25 percent and 50 percent. The remainder is equally divided between unskilled and unemployed workers. We also assume that a 1 percent increase in the prevalence level can be associated with a 0 to 1 percent reduction in total factor productivity. This is below the range suggested by other studies in the literature in which the impact is more in the 0.5 to 1 percent range (see, for example, Haacker [2001] and MacFarlan and Sgherri [2001]).

9. The present value simply puts future production and consumption into today's monetary equivalents. For instance, if banks pay a 5 percent interest rate per year, US$105 12 months from now is equivalent to US$100 today.

10. As a reference, in Thailand, the reduction in the population growth rate resulting from the epidemic has been estimated at 0.1 percent per year, while, in Botswana, it reaches 2.5 percent per year. On average, estimates in the literature predict a 1 percentage point reduction in the population growth rate.

11. For instance, if in a given population, low-income individuals die as a result of the epidemic, the average income of the remaining workers will increase even if their individual income remains constant. The epidemic would appear to have a positive effect on average.

12. These calculations are based on the baseline total population in the absence of HIV/AIDS.

CHAPTER 5

Responses to
HIV/AIDS

The MENA/EM countries are currently at the crossroads in their response to HIV/AIDS, with a growing number having recently initiated a more comprehensive planning process aimed at implementing locally adapted, effective, and sustained actions to deal with the epidemic. Until 1999 and 2000, the response to HIV/AIDS had been largely limited to actions taken in the health sector, including the training of health care workers, AIDS case reporting and surveillance, and infection control and blood safety, but HIV/AIDS had not yet been recognized as a leading public health, social, and development concern. Although many countries initiated HIV/AIDS awareness-raising activities early on, limited information and capacity currently exists to address such key issues as provision of prevention and care among young people and reaching vulnerable and at-risk groups.

In many countries, HIV/AIDS prevention, care, and support services are mostly provided through the NAPs of the ministries of health, with, as yet, insufficient involvement of other sectors and civil society actors. However, NGOs now play an essential role in Algeria, Djibouti, Lebanon, Morocco, Sudan, and Tunisia, and in a few countries PLWHA have become key partners in the response. The NAPs, themselves, remain, with a few exceptions, understaffed and urgently need to strengthen their human capacities at the central and peripheral levels. The public budget allocated to NAPs in many countries remains insufficient to cover the normative functions of the program, let alone ensure an intensification and expansion of actions. Since 1996, many of the NAPs have relied on specific program funding through UNAIDS, WHO, UNICEF, UNFPA, the United Nations Development Programme (UNDP), the World Bank, and bilateral partners to carry out essential surveillance, prevention, care, and support actions.

Over the past two years, an increased number of countries have initiated strategic planning on HIV/AIDS, involving both the health and nonhealth sectors. Egypt, Jordan, Lebanon, Somalia, and Syria are some of the countries now planning or conducting a situation-and-response assessment on HIV/AIDS, while Algeria, Djibouti, the Islamic Republic of Iran, Morocco, the Republic of Yemen, and Sudan are among the countries that have already formulated their strategic frameworks. It is expected that these plans will lead to sustained HIV/AIDS actions in a range of sectors, such as education, religious affairs, young people, labor, media, uniformed services, and prison systems.

National Health Systems

No single indicator can predict the spread of HIV, but the interaction of different factors produces scenarios of likelihood. The state of public health services, however, may be considered a sound predictor of the capacity of a nation to handle the considerable health consequences of HIV. Over the past 30 years, the MENA/EM region's highly centralized governments have taken the responsibility for economic and social development. The development of health services has often focused on the expansion of infrastructure over concerns for quality, efficiency, and sustainability. The inability of the public sector to secure sufficient funding or offer quality services has encouraged the expansion of private sector services, but these services remain largely unregulated. From proper laboratory testing for HIV as part of surveillance and case detection, universal precautions in all health facilities, hospital waste management, safe injecting and safe blood supplies, STI diagnosis and treatment, voluntary counseling and testing (VCT), and mass public health education, to HIV treatment (both care of opportunistic infections and antiretroviral therapy [ART]), the capacity to meet requirements is questionable on at least a few counts even in the best health care systems. Prevention of mother-to-child transmission (MTCT) with the use of antiretrovirals, such as AZT (zidovudine) or nevirapine for example, requires the capacity to screen, counsel, administer the drugs properly, monitor their effects, handle any complications, manage issues of breastfeeding versus bottle-feeding, and follow up on the pediatric issues associated with infected and noninfected children. In countries such as Oman, with modern medical facilities, these needs may be met, but across the region issues of confidentiality and stigma continue to cause patients to seek care privately or in other countries. In countries with poorer health systems, overall capacity ranges from low to totally lacking. Among Libyans, for example, it is reported that many go to Tunisia to seek care, presumably through the private sector.

Blood safety is universally established (except in the Republic of Yemen), but in some nations cannot be considered thoroughly safe. Because of the generally low prevalence of HIV, a lack of awareness of the seriousness of other blood-borne viruses, and confidence in the protectiveness of social norms, universal precautions are officially adopted but often not followed.

It is said that VCT is available in many countries, yet, although testing is available, it is not always accompanied by pre- and posttest counseling.

STD services within the public health system vary widely from poor, as in Djibouti and the Republic of Yemen, to a widespread attempt to improve STD services, as in Morocco. In Tunisia's youth program, there appears to have been an effort to make STD services both accessible and friendly to young people. Some efforts have been made in Egypt's reproductive health programs to teach village midwives about HIV, but the information given to date has been limited.

In a growing number of countries, for example, Algeria, Bahrain, the Islamic Republic of Iran, Jordan, Lebanon, Morocco, Oman, and Tunisia, ART is either available or may soon be available through the public sector on a limited basis. This is an expensive option, and Tunisia had estimated that, at the prices available at the time, giving triple drug therapy to an estimated 250 persons by the end of 2001 will use 95 percent of the Ministry of Health HIV/AIDS budget (Ben Said 2001a).

Algeria is similarly supplying free ART to several hundred people. Efforts are under way to negotiate bulk purchases and identify alternate drug suppliers, and prices are changing rapidly. In the countries mentioned above, as well as Syria, AZT is available to infected antenatal patients to diminish perinatal transmission. The Accelerated Access to Care Initiative supported by UNAIDS/WHO and other partners is now contributing to negotiations with pharmaceutical firms in a number of countries, such as Lebanon, Morocco, and Tunisia (WHO/EMRO 2003). No discussion regarding breastfeeding policies was documented for any countries.

The management of opportunistic infections and general health care for HIV-infected people is severely hampered by the negative attitudes of health providers, lack of drugs and supplies, and dysfunctional health systems where these exist in the region. In some nations, people found to be infected are sent to a person associated with the NAP for counseling because specifically trained HIV counselors are not widely available. In Algeria, Djibouti, Egypt, Jordan, and Morocco, numerous counselors have been trained but there has been no evaluation of their functioning or effectiveness. In Egypt, infected people are managed through the "fever" hospitals. Oman appears to have developed a facility-based system of treatment, care, and counseling. In the Republic of Yemen, neither private nor public facilities as yet appear ready to manage patients with HIV (see box 5.1).

Efforts to diminish HIV-associated stigma and discrimination in the general population have been minimal and are not widespread. More

BOX 5.1

Situation and Needs Assessment in the Republic of Yemen

Geographic access to public health facilities remains limited, with only 30 percent of the rural population having access to health care and only 50 percent access overall. However, real access—as measured by the presence of services within present health facilities—is substantially lower. Even where facilities are available, their utilization appears to be low. Because of the lack of essential drugs and services in government health facilities, a bypass rate of 42 to 73 percent has been found. The total expenditure on health in the Republic of Yemen remains among the lowest in the Middle East region, accounting for just 1.1 percent of GDP in 1998. Actual government health expenditure per capita is US$2.58, compared with a benchmark ideal of US$12.

In a survey of health care workers, the majority of respondents believed that AIDS patients should be isolated and receive care in specialized hospitals. More than two-thirds of respondents refused to give care to HIV-positive people or AIDS patients. Among the reasons were the possibility of infection transmission to other patients and absence of preventive tools. Eighty percent of all respondents reported accidental pricks during work, and half of them would go and clean the site of prick. Ninety-two percent of respondents were unaware of any guideline or protocol for care or support for HIV-positive people or AIDS patients. Fifty percent of all the health care personnel have never had any in-service training of any form, and 67 percent never had any kind of training on HIV/AIDS.

All of the visited sites had laboratory facilities. The use of gloves while handling blood and blood samples was not common in all the observed facilities. In one of the hospitals, none of the technicians were using gloves. In two of the facilities, technicians were still using mouth pipettes. There appears to be a 50 percent gap between the actual need for gloves and medical supplies and what is available. A special box for sharp instruments and needles was observed in only one facility. In other facilities, technicians were using an ordinary dustbin (woven, side holes) for disposal of needles and sharp instruments. All of the facilities were disposing their waste through an unqualified private company, which collected the waste without any safety measures for the handling of hospital waste and took it to the same place where the city waste is disposed.

Sometimes, extreme measures have been taken. In one hospital, after finding an HIV-positive patient in the surgical ward, they burned all the belongings and closed that room for five days. Only one facility admits known HIV/AIDS patients, and those patients are put in isolation.

Source: UNAIDS 2000.

often, training has been conducted for health workers that is aimed at diminishing their fear of handling HIV patients. Media (print and TV) continue to produce stories on HIV/AIDS that negatively influence popular opinion in some countries. In Egypt, efforts have been made by the NAP, through UNICEF support, to educate media personnel. Building on a powerful media sector, as in Egypt, Lebanon, and the Gulf states, U.N. agencies have embarked on a regional initiative in 2003 to increase the contribution of media to HIV/AIDS awareness beyond their regular interventions made around World AIDS Day. Overall, governments have made few efforts to address stigma and discrimination.

Other Sectors

While different sectors of government sit on national AIDS committees, substantive programs initiated by sectors other than health, for example, education, remain relatively recent in the region. The United Nations Educational, Scientific, and Cultural Organization (UNESCO) undertook a consultation in 2001 that brought together representatives of the ministries of health and of education from the countries in the region to review and plan for greater integration of HIV/AIDS into educational curricula (UNESCO/UNAIDS 2001). In Morocco, the new national strategic plan includes significant activities for the ministries of education, justice (prisons), and youth and sports (rural young). In most other countries, such as Jordan and Egypt, HIV/AIDS education has been conducted in school settings on a one-off basis and with limited coverage. Egypt does have a component of the high school curriculum that covers reproductive health, but there is evidence that it is not very effective.

Algeria, Djibouti, the Islamic Republic of Iran, the Republic of Yemen, and Sudan are or have also recently developed planning for different sectors, including education, young people, religious affairs, media, labor, uniformed services, and so forth, as part of a larger effort aimed at addressing factors of risk and vulnerability and the consequences of the epidemic. However, implementation to date remains limited to selected interventions funded through national resources, U.N. agencies, and other partners.

In several countries, government sectors other than health are involved in drug control and the rehabilitation of drug-dependent people. Demand reduction for drug use has been promoted in the region, though the concept of harm reduction has only been recently introduced, making it unlikely to affect IDU rates in the short run. Most countries operate inpatient drug detoxification treatment facilities at one or a few hospitals; a few countries have outpatient care as well. None has drug-substitution programs or allow needle/syringe distribution, except the Islamic Republic of Iran. Research results have apparently driven increased political commitment in recent years, and considerable openness about the problem is evidenced in local newspapers. The Islamic Republic of Iran has embarked on a broad-based approach to drug demand reduction, drug treatment, and harm reduction with the support of UNODC and other agencies. The Welfare Organization and the Justice Department work directly with the Ministry of Health (MoH) on drug-related issues, a portion of which include HIV (see box 5.2).

International and Local Nongovernmental Organizations

In addition to inadequate surveillance throughout the region, there are few targeted interventions, including risk-reduction approaches, for specific groups, such as in Lebanon. Cooperation with INGOs, local NGOS, or community-based organizations (CBOs) is generally halting. In only a few nations (Algeria, Djibouti, and Sudan), progress has been made in developing collaborative relations between government and organizations representing PLWHA, although there appears to be a growing recognition that this effort should take place. Recently, there has been positive progress in mobilizing national NGOs at both country and regional levels in the response to HIV/AIDS. A regional network of NGOs on HIV/AIDS was established in December 2002 through the support of the UNDP HIV/AIDS Regional Program for Arab States and UNAIDS. The regional network will aim to mobilize the active participation of NGOs in the country response and strengthen their capacities to implement HIV/AIDS activities. Youth have been the target of a significant intervention in Tunisia (see box 5.3) as well as in other countries such as Jordan, Oman, and Syria (Ministry of Health, Jordan 1999; Ministry of Health, Sultanate of Oman, 2000; Ministry of Health, Syrian Arab Republic 2000).

More general reproductive health programs are found in most countries, executed both through the government health services and with some NGOs. These programs have been slow, however, to incorporate HIV/AIDS issues into their activities.

Foundations such as Ford Foundation and INGOs such as the Population Council, Family Health International, and Save the Children have conducted important related research and contribute to the overall effort at improved sexual and reproductive health. In Egypt, the Ford Foundation and other partners fund the government hotline in Cairo.

BOX 5.2

VCT and Harm-Reduction Programs in the Islamic Republic of Iran

In 1999, a large VCT program was started, with each urban district having at least one VCT center. In addition to the VCT services provided by 85 blood banks, there are now VCT centers in health centers run by the MoH and in rehabilitation centers run by the Welfare Organization and the Justice Department. VCT services are provided according to MoH guidelines. Counseling is provided by psychologists, psychiatrists, general practitioners, and other heath care workers who have been specifically trained for this purpose. The MoH provides training for the counselors. HIV tests are performed in the laboratories of the blood transfusion organization. Sera are screened by two different enzyme-linked immunosorbent assay (ELISA) tests, and ELISA-positive sera are confirmed by Western blot.

All VCT services are provided free of charge. Most clients come directly on their own initiative, while others are referred, including family members of both IDUs and HIV-positive individuals. Referred clients who do not report any risk or risky behavior for themselves are advised that they do not need an HIV test. However, any client who wishes to take a test can do so. In 18 months, more than 75,000 clients have been counseled at the VCT centers, and more than 61,000 clients have been tested.

The harm-reduction program in the Islamic Republic of Iran is recent. It was started in 2000 in the capitals of the three provinces that are most affected by injecting drug use (Kermanshah, Shiraz, and Tehran). It is a pilot project initiated by the MoH working with locally based physicians and volunteers. The harm-reduction services are provided in outpatient clinics. These clinics also provide services for HIV-positive patients (counseling, clinical management including antiretrovirals, laboratory tests, and social support), as well as education, counseling, and management of STIs. All services are free of charge and confidential. IDUs are provided counseling, methadone treatment, and needle exchange. For example, the clinic in Kermanshah sees 700 clients per month, most of them HIV-positive individuals and their family members. About 150 clients are on methadone, and about 50 come for the needle exchange. Initial reactions are positive, both from the staff and clients. In mid-2001, the results of the pilot program were presented to the cabinet and the president. On the basis of the initial results, the continuation and expansion of the program were approved.

Source: U.S. Census Bureau 2001.

Care and support, including home-based care, for those infected with HIV are usually best provided by NGOs. Relatively few support groups formed of HIV-positive people have developed in the region, although such group support is becoming more regular in Lebanon, the Islamic Republic of Iran, and other countries. In Djibouti and the Republic of Yemen, INGO-run clinics appear to offer the most effective care for the

---

BOX 5.3

Tunisia: Youth and Condoms

Tunisia is one nation in the region that has begun to conceptualize and carry out large interventions among youth. Tunisia developed modern approaches to gender equity within a context of Islamic traditions decades ago. Nearly equal proportions of males and females complete secondary school (44.2 percent males versus 47.3 percent females) and tertiary education (9.6 percent males versus 6.9 percent females) and know about contraception (83.4 percent males versus 79.3 percent females) and STDs (84 percent males versus 75.4 percent females). The current average age at marriage is 30 for males and 26 for females, although young people themselves wish it were earlier, at about 27 for males and 22 for females. Few marriages are arranged, and young people have considerable personal mobility. Recognizing the vulnerability of young people, who are facing unemployment rates twice that of the general population (30 percent versus 16 percent) and the lack of sexual/reproductive educational or health services specifically designed for the young, UNFPA, in collaboration with the Department of the Family and Population, began a program in late 1997 designed to reach 10 percent of the 85,000 youth between 15 and 24 years old in the nation. Regional and provincial counseling centers for youth were set up, including some in student dormitories, on school campuses, and at factories and trade schools. Several NGOs participated, including the Arab Scouts, Médecins sans Frontières, and the IPPF.

In addition to providing confidential counseling, STI screening and treatment, abortion, and contraceptives, the project has distributed 2 million condoms since 1998. There were constraints related to how and where the condoms could be distributed, but some creative maneuvering placed them into easily accessible dispenser boxes outside of medical service offices at the schools and dormitories. Students can simply take what they wish without asking anyone. Recently, the installation of condom vending machines at universities has been considered. The project has been evaluated, and the next phase is in the process of being planned.

Source: Ben Yahia 2000; Gueddána and others 1996; Ministry of Public Health, Tunisia 2000.

---

poorer segments of the population. In the Republic of Yemen, this care is for STDs only and not for HIV.

Where local NGOs have not been developed or are not well supported by government policies, it will be extremely difficult for government agencies themselves to reach the most needy people. It is unlikely that local NGOs, where they exist, would take up HIV/AIDS work unless they receive government blessings for the task.

Private Sector

No documentation has revealed any involvement of the private sector. This apparent lack of involvement may be because almost all documentation is produced by the various MoHs. It is more likely, however, that like NGOs, private companies would not involve themselves with a stigmatized disease unless governments led the way and included the private sector in a truly multilateral approach.

United Nations Agencies

U.N. agencies have played an important role in most countries in the region over the past 15 years. The U.N. agencies and other key partners have recently substantially increased their commitment to HIV/AIDS in the region. In the first Regional Meeting of UNAIDS Cosponsors and Key Partners on HIV/AIDS, held in Cairo in November 2001, the regional priorities on HIV/AIDS were defined (UNAIDS 2001). Since then, the U.N. agencies have increased their resources and expanded their activities on HIV/AIDS. Currently, they are developing their strategic vision and action plans in their programmatic areas of work on HIV/AIDS, strengthening their human capacities, and supporting country-based activities.

WHO/EMRO has advocated for improved serosurveillance, STI diagnosis and treatment, heightened awareness of vulnerability, and improved national programs by convening regional meetings and providing technical assistance on specific missions. In a recent effort to improve the response of the region's health sectors, WHO/EMRO has drafted a strategy, set goals, and suggested approaches to meet those goals. The strategy includes the following targets to be attained between 2003 and 2005:

- Improve political commitment and public information about HIV/AIDS.

- Improve institutional mechanisms and capacity to deal with HIV/AIDS and STD prevention and care.

- Integrate packages of HIV/AIDS and STD prevention and care into the health-delivery systems.

- Improve the capacity to generate relevant information and apply operational research to the problems of HIV/AIDS and STDs.

- Incorporate HIV/AIDS and STD prevention and care into national responses to complex emergencies, including conflicts, population displacement, and embargoes.

UNODC has initiated a national assessment of drug-use patterns in a few countries and the integration of HIV/AIDS into their prevention programs for young people. A recent desk review, commissioned by UNODC, of drug-abuse problems throughout the region inventories the more accessible information on drug-treatment services but reveals the paucity of clear, up-to-date information on practices among users (Groterath and Bless 2002). UNESCO is focusing on HIV/AIDS preventive education, and the International Labour Organisation is initiating activities addressing HIV/AIDS in the world of work. UNDP is currently implementing the HIV/AIDS Regional Program for Arab States, focusing on support for NGOs, PLWHA, media, human rights, and gender issues. UNICEF and UNFPA are addressing prevention among young people and selected vulnerable groups, initiating prevention of MTCT in a few countries in the region and VCT services in collaboration with WHO/EMRO. Condom provision has been largely supported through UNFPA. The World Bank has incorporated assessments of the HIV/AIDS situation into health project preparations for several countries, offered funds for such assessments to others, and is financing a large HIV/AIDS project in Djibouti. Improving responses from national financial sectors to mitigate the extensive economic aspects of HIV has not been emphasized in the past, but it is a goal the Bank is in a strong position to promote in the future.

The UNAIDS Unified Budget and Workplan for HIV/AIDS has facilitated the acquisition of increasing levels of funds for most of the agencies, most notably for UNICEF, UNDP, UNFPA, UNESCO, the International Labour Organisation, and UNODC.

The role of UNAIDS in the region has increased over the past years in support of mobilizing and strengthening HIV/AIDS response at regional and country levels. At the regional level, UNAIDS has assisted agencies to develop their strategic thinking on HIV/AIDS, leverage resources, and facilitate coordination across different partners. At the country level, UNAIDS has focused its support to situation assessments on the determinants of vulnerability, strategic planning across sectors, and capacity building in implementation, with emphasis on vulnerable groups, young people, and other priority areas of work. In an effort to advance the response, plans exist to facilitate the efforts of cosponsors and other stakeholders by:

- Supporting situation assessments, strategic planning, and program development that focuses on the determinants, risks, and consequences of HIV/AIDS.

- Facilitating coordination at the regional and national levels between UNAIDS cosponsors and other partners in strategy development, integrated planning, and strategic information on the response.

- Mobilizing awareness and human and financial resources of partners.

- Building networks of resource people, NGOs, and institutions working in priority areas of the HIV/AIDS response.

- Mobilizing support for the exchange of experiences, information sharing, and documentation of best practices on the basis of country needs.

- Developing capacities to reach vulnerable populations through appropriate approaches.

UNAIDS channels its support to country activities through the Theme Groups (TGs) on HIV/AIDS, which have been established since 1996.

In nearly all countries of the region, national AIDS committees or NAPs were established by the late 1980s or early 1990s. Of the current 15 Theme Groups on HIV/AIDS in the 20 countries this review covers, some are functional but have not taken much collective action, and others provide generally effective forums for decisionmaking and coordination. However, in the past year, an increased number of Theme Groups have become more active entities with a wider participation of country-based actors. Despite the positive developments described above, there is an urgent need to reinforce coordination between key stakeholders in all countries in the region. Most countries have not yet engaged in a full policy process, although in some, such as Tunisia, there appears to be strong political commitment despite relatively low levels of investment.

Bilateral Donors

Bilateral donors, such as USAID, have carried out specific research or assessment tasks and invested in specific projects such as training counselors in Jordan and supporting the hotline, improving blood donation systems, and training health workers in Egypt. The Swiss government has aided Egypt in developing an advanced blood safety system. The French government has played a large role in Djibouti, but its own recent evaluation pointed to inadequate effectiveness; thus, new plans are under way to alter activities, which will include the building of a new facility specifically for treatment of STIs.

Overall, the response to HIV/AIDS in the region has been slow and has concentrated on extensive mandatory testing, medical issues such as blood supply safety, and, increasingly, on treatment of AIDS patients. The social and economic factors that drive an HIV epidemic have not been addressed, either with research or interventions. Issues associated with youth form the one exception to this generalization but, to date, have been inadequate to make an impact in almost all nations. Political leaders have not viewed HIV as an important issue for their countries, with the recent exception of Djibouti, Morocco, Sudan and, earlier, Tunisia. Small AIDS program budgets significantly constrain activities in most nations. The overwhelmingly dominant role of the MoHs in the response so far underscores a narrow view in the region of HIV as a medical issue. Advocacy for collaborative multisectoral activities is essential, as are concrete plans for moving such an effort forward.

Little coordination of efforts among donors further constrains both planning and action. A thorough revitalization of commitment is urgently needed, a move we hope will be promoted through dialogue facilitated by this book.

CHAPTER 6

A Way Forward

Raising the Priority of HIV/AIDS

The potential strength of a broadly collaborative effort to diminish HIV risk, vulnerability, and impact has yet to be developed in the region. National governments can develop such a comprehensive response in collaboration with U.N. agencies, bilateral donors, and local actors.

Political, cultural, and capacity-related barriers, in addition to the apparent low HIV prevalence, have continued to push HIV prevention and care to a low priority level. Some political leaders have yet to be convinced that increased investment is essential. While still underused in other areas, expressive performances, including documentaries, have yet to emerge in the MENA/EM region, though these were clearly effective in awakening political concern in some nations, for example, in India. Effective, coordinated planning and action across government ministries is rare, and the additional essential involvement of NGOs is rarer still. In Algeria, Djibouti, Morocco, and Sudan, intensified plans of action are being developed with steps taken to ensure coordination across several governmental domains. Elsewhere, where increased commitment and investment has not yet taken place, research into the actual risks of spread and vulnerabilities must be undertaken and used for advocacy, in order to achieve greater investment.

Where overall HIV prevalence is low, it is usual for leaders to stall and postpone, waiting for increased outbreaks. In country after country, this has been shown to be an unwise and high-risk strategy. Reviews conducted by the World Bank in 1997 clearly showed that the cost of investing when the epidemic was not yet widespread is far less than the losses accrued when rates of HIV rise (World Bank 1999a). Senegal and Bangladesh are two of a small number of nations with low prevalence rates that invested in full country programs early, and have had much success to date in keeping prevalence levels low. In the MENA/EM region, Algeria, the Islamic Republic of Iran, Lebanon, and Morocco appear to be the next examples of low-prevalence nations that are ready to develop and carry out substantial prevention programs. Morocco provides a further example of the success of a strategic planning process in which all stakeholders have a part (see box 6.1).

Algeria has engaged in a similar process of developing its strategic plan on HIV/AIDS across sectors with wide participation of different ministries, NGOs, and international partners. The Islamic Republic of Iran has, to date, focused on the risk from drug use, and, as yet, has little involvement of NGOs. It will certainly need to include sex workers and others quickly, a task that, in most countries, is best carried out by NGOs in collaboration with government. In all of these examples, credible and useful research had taken place to inform decisionmakers. The production of that knowledge was not for academic papers or media consumption, but for those with legitimate interests in HIV prevention such as government bodies, NGOs, donors, and others. Djibouti, on the other

---

BOX 6.1

Strategic Planning for HIV/AIDS in Morocco

The process of developing a strategic plan for Morocco began by drafting a report analyzing the situation and the national response to HIV/AIDS. This process dealt with the epidemiological situation and its evolution, the formation of earlier national plans, and the actual responses that were implemented in relation to the aims of those plans. In addition, the report sought to assess the human and financial resources available in the fight against HIV/AIDS. Special sections were devoted to reports on the regions of Tanger, Agadir, and Marrakech. Specific chapters analyzed the situation with respect to the impact on the individual, the family, and society; the patterns of drug use, systems of sex work, and gender roles in Moroccan society; and the responses of the NGO sector. There also was a synthesis of the regional responses and an analysis of overall obstacles and opportunities.

Workshops to develop local plans took place in the regions of Tanger, Agadir, and Marrakech. A three-day National Consensus Workshop was held in Rabat with a wide range of invited participants, including different government ministries, all NGOs able to contribute to AIDS-related work, the U.N. Theme Group members, and potential donors. Carefully prepared beforehand, seven presentations were made and eight facilitators were retained to lead the process of attaining consensus from participants. The result is a comprehensive, budgeted program formulated on the basis of a range of available information, the principles of social development, and clear definitions of roles across several government offices, NGOs, and other stakeholders.

Source: Farza 2001.

hand, is a country that, despite having conducted enough research to demonstrate risk factors, waited too long and now has a generalized epidemic that will require a great deal of investment to reduce its impact.

A program of solid sociobehavioral research is needed in most countries to establish the types, contexts, and determinants of high-risk behaviors wherever they take place, identify those groups that may engage in such behaviors at higher frequencies than others, estimate the sizes of such groups, design appropriate interventions, and monitor the impact of prevention and care programs among them.

This process requires a thorough review of all published and unpublished materials, including master's and doctoral theses. In most countries, there are researchers who have worked on reproductive health issues or even family planning. With some help, perhaps even support and training from the well-known programs of the Ford Foundation, these people can be enlisted to develop new research on gender and sexuality issues, building on the substantial foundation already present in the region (Al-Jowder 2001; Davis 1992; Davis and Davis 1989; El-Tawila 2000; Ghannam 1997; Ghurayyib 1992; Ilkkaracen 2000; Khattab 1996; Mernissi 2000; Murray and Roscoe 1997; Obermeyer 1994, 2000; Reysoo 1999; Schmitt and Sofer 1992; Seif El Dawla, Abdel Hadi, and Abdel Wahab 1998; Shabaan 2000; Shokrollahi and others 1999; Von Bruck 1997; Wikan 1976).

Specific recommendations for the related domains of research and policy are as follows:

- Formative studies should be qualitative and ethnographic, followed by quantitative surveys after a rapport is developed and trust is ensured. It is important that researchers use the information gained to enlighten decisionmakers in a manner that encourages humane understanding and nonpunitive interventions.

- A valuable approach to raising the priority of HIV/AIDS is to initiate a full policy development process, one that includes the participation of many stakeholders and evolves over a limited time into a consensus of needed actions.

- The development of policy has many functions and provides a template on which actions can be planned. One of the most important aspects of the making of an HIV/AIDS policy is the process by which all stakeholders are given a chance to debate, discuss, and come to some agreement on the steps that can be taken to advance HIV/AIDS prevention and care in each country. While such a process can take a year or more, it is well worth the effort if it results in raising the awareness of key people in specific ministries who have a role in reducing vulnerability. Furthermore, it can set out areas in which research is required and legitimize research efforts that might otherwise be considered too sensitive.

Reaching Hidden Populations

The sensitivities of countries in the MENA/EM region to public statements concerning socially and religiously disapproved groups were quite apparent at the United Nations General Assembly Special Session on HIV/AIDS (UNGASS) held in New York in mid-2001. Strong religious and social disapproval may, in fact, deter some people from engaging in behavior that is both risky and viewed as immoral, but it is profoundly false to claim there is *no* risk. Even small levels of risk, that is, small groups of people involved in high-risk activities, can form the core of transmission for a nation. This is certainly true in Indonesia, where it has taken more than a decade for the epidemic to become clearly visible.

For that reason, special and unobtrusive methods must be used to reach socially and legally marginalized groups. This effort is possible if political arrangements can be made between concerned agencies, and if a trusted INGO or local NGO is given permission to do so. In Morocco and Bangladesh, MSM have been successfully reached in this way (see box 6.2).

Specifically, reaching hidden populations can be accomplished in a variety of ways. Some suggestions are as follows:

- Reproductive health programs can reach sex workers in a variety of unobtrusive ways, such as by setting up a neighborhood clinic for disadvantaged women or simply for local women, and letting it be known that specially trained and sympathetic staff are available who understand the needs of sex workers. In Vietnam, small women's health clubs are serving this purpose. Alternatively, outreach workers can reach women at night and show them a site they could access in the daytime for information and services. Inside the site, either a real clinic front or a private apartment or house, a small clinic could be set up for STD diagnosis and treatment. Exploratory ethnographic research would be required to fit the service to the situation and must closely involve members of the at-risk community. Alternative methods of reaching hidden groups have been used in many countries.

- One important approach is to develop specific HIV prevention programs for policemen or security forces and their wives. Once the barrier is broken in discussing prevention issues with these men, it is often much easier to gain cooperation for outreach programs on the

---

BOX 6.2

Reaching MSM in Morocco and Bangladesh

In Morocco, the Moroccan AIDS Service Organization (Association Marocaine de Lutte contre le SIDA), a voluntary organization led by a well-known woman doctor, undertook a small action research project with male sex workers in 1993. Aware that these are highly marginalized people and that homosexuality is a crime punishable by three to six months in prison, the organization proceeded cautiously, building its intervention around peer education and outreach. One of the greatest obstacles was the police because they interpreted the possession of condoms as evidence of sex work, which led to many men not wanting to have condoms with them. The organization set up safe spaces for discussion groups, distributed condoms and information brochures, and provided referrals for voluntary counseling and testing. The project is continuing in the context of a wider set of projects for marginalized groups in Morocco.

In Bangladesh, the Bandhu Social Welfare Society began its work in 1998. With careful documentation, advocacy with local police, quiet explanations to national AIDS authorities, and presentations to donors, its work has become quite appreciated, despite the taboo that continues to surround male-to-male sex. With access to men through Bandhu's STD clinics, the NAP has been able to include samples of both male sex workers and MSM who do not sell sex in the annual sentinel surveillance for HIV and syphilis. The behavioral surveillance also includes the same groups, randomly sampled in the city of Dhaka, and has been extended, along with an intervention, to include *hijras*, South Asia's transgender population. In the second year of surveillance, the success of the intervention was statistically demonstrated, convincing donors to invest in its expansion. HIV prevalence remains low in this group, and syphilis rates appear to be dropping. Since 2000, the NAP has also been a donor, helping Bandhu to reach male sex workers in other cities of Bangladesh. The Bandhu Social Welfare Society has taken a lead role in important research concerning masculinity and male sexual and reproductive responsibility and has become one of the major players in the national response. One key to success has been its leaders, who are respectful, religious, and committed young men.

Source: Boushaba and Hammich 2000; Boushaba and others 1999; Jenkins, Ahmed, and others 2001.

---

streets and in public places to people who might be subject to arrest for sex work or drug use. Even without a formal intervention for police, repeated closed-door discussions can play an important role in HIV advocacy and prevention. Similar processes are essential for other uniformed personnel such as military troops, border patrol officers, and others.

- IDUs seem to be somewhat less stigmatized in the MENA/EM region than sex-related risk groups. Hence, reaching out to IDUs can be done in a more institutionalized fashion, but may require amendments to specific laws. Again, a thorough policy review is needed to harmonize drug-control and HIV-prevention strategies and approaches. The Islamic Republic of Iran has exemplified the way forward for the region with regard to IDUs and HIV risk.

Reducing the Vulnerability of Migrants

HIV prevention among migrants is an international issue. Coordinated programs between host and sender countries are essential, and they must develop beyond the mere screening that takes place at present. Through the existing frameworks of agreement between IOM and UNHCR with UNAIDS, these agencies' participation is essential. The UNAIDS Secretariat and the concerned agencies should take the lead in planning and coordinating prevention initiatives for migrants in the MENA/EM region and advocate at any forum that has political or economic reach across the region.

IOM has developed specific programs in collaboration with host governments for migrants in difficult circumstances. Most recently, such a program was implemented for Burmese migrants in northern Thailand. The methods by which this program was negotiated require some review and probable adaptation, but do provide an example in which disadvantaged foreigners can gain access to needed information and services. Furthermore, where temporary migration across borders, as in Algeria, appears to be the main concern, the new Mekong regional program, which has demonstrated behavioral surveillance among border crossers, could serve as an example. An older, well-known example of cross-border HIV prevention through outreach and clinic services operates at the Nepalese-Indian border. This program has been documented and evaluated, although no surveillance has taken place in the associated subpopulation groups.

UNHCR and UNAIDS have specific roles in negotiating HIV prevention and care for refugees, whose rights in host countries need protection. In the MENA/EM region, the rights of refugees in the Republic of Yemen to gain access to information, VCT, STD services, and care and support will not be honored unless the same services are set up for Yemeni citizens. This step has yet to take place.

HIV prevention among tourists has many precedents. Australia, in particular, has developed a set of well-known strategies appropriate for Australian travelers in Asia. In the Maldives, the national association of tourism instituted HIV-prevention training in the tourist workers' pre-professional training schools and pledged to install condom vending machines in hotels, which has value for both tourists and local workers. Condom vending machines are particularly acceptable in scenarios of anonymity and commerce. Thailand is developing a program to install them in universities.

Providing Practical Information and Means of Prevention

Little is known about the level of knowledge of HIV in the region. One study in Jordan seemed to indicate that levels of knowledge have dropped in recent years. Mass media engagement in educating the public has not been fully used, and most efforts have been small and face to face. When, however, films or plays have been used, as in Lebanon, Oman, and recently in the Republic of Yemen, these have considerable success at mobilizing public concern. If a population only hears about HIV/AIDS on World AIDS Day, it is likely that many citizens would not believe HIV could be a threat to the public. The first generation of AIDS information, that is, modes of transmission, is still not widely and correctly understood. Although knowledge does not in itself alter behavior, it is a prerequisite for both personally initiated behavior change and the participation of civil society in joining a national effort for HIV prevention.

Sensitivities about condoms have proved to be a major barrier in the MENA/EM region. As there are not yet any other devices that can prevent the spread of HIV through sexual contact, educating people about the modes of transmission without making the means of prevention either known or available can hardly be considered adequate public health action. The frequently documented lack of condom education and distribution to STD patients by health providers in the region is clearly unethical. The fear associated with promotion of condoms in conservative societies has not proved to be well founded. Where behavioral surveillance has been able to track sexual behaviors among specific population groups, for example, taxi drivers or truck drivers, government promotion of condoms did not lead to increased sexual activity. In fact, in most cases, the incidence of illicit sex dropped and condom use increased at the same time (Family Health International 2001a).

Some suggested steps for the MENA/EM region are as follows:

- The much-needed debate about how to increase awareness and distribution of condoms is best done in a forum of stakeholders gathered together as part of a policy process. Small steps can be taken and monitored. Religious leaders can play an important role by advocating for behaviors in line with morality, but people have the right to condoms to protect themselves from a fatal disease in the same way a child has the right to a measles vaccine. The two approaches are not incompatible, as has been seen in Bangladesh, Indonesia, Senegal, Uganda, and other conservative societies.

- Female condoms are increasingly found to provide options to women in many countries and circumstances. Reproductive health programs could begin to explore the acceptability of the female condom, as is planned in Tunisia.

Reducing the Vulnerability of Youth

It is clear that reproductive health for young people is both a sensitive and important issue, which elicits considerable concern in the region. Multisectoral planning is of value in this arena, as educational authorities, labor regulation agencies, and planning offices should be considering the impact of economic policies on the cost of education, access to employment, and alleviation of the pressures on unemployed young men and women. Drug demand–reduction education should also be included in a multisectoral effort for the region's youth.

There is considerable scope to develop culturally appropriate "life skills" educational programs specifically for young people, both in and out of school settings. UNICEF, UNESCO, and many others have developed excellent packages for youth in a wide variety of societies. Proper formative research is required, and a professional process of developing such programs is essential.

Care and Support

There is a need to increase provision of care and counseling, including psychosocial support for the HIV/AIDS infected and affected, and to evaluate the ongoing programs in the region. Ongoing studies of the quality of services, from the point of view of the clients and the caregivers, are essential. No programs for the care of orphans have been clarified. Most important, little has been done to reduce stigma and discrimination on a popular level in most countries. The success of both prevention and care projects depends to a large extent on the degree of community acceptance and mobilization. This effort may require additional services, such as income generation and legal services. A wider view of care and support will become increasingly necessary as the number of AIDS cases grows. Home-based care will be needed. This is particularly true in Djibouti, Somalia, and Sudan.

But even where those with AIDS will receive ART, prevention counseling, including outreach programs, cannot be dispensed with. Country program managers and HIV-infected people alike should guard against viewing the administration of ART as *the* solution to the problem of HIV/AIDS. The network of NGOs on HIV/AIDS recently established in the region should strengthen the capacities of NGOs and increase their involvement in the implementation of HIV/AIDS interventions, with a particular focus on vulnerable and at-risk groups.

Structural Factors

Improving health care systems, developing greater access to information for the public, and working with INGOs and NGOs to accomplish national goals are all issues that require policy discussions with a broad-based coalition of partners in change.

Multisectoral planning may be best led by a national planning committee rather than a health department. HIV is not simply a disease; it is a plague that follows the cracks in unstable or inadequate systems and mirrors the human development conditions in a nation.

Working with Communities

Where only the government holds the power to make decisions, gain and utilize resources, and carry out the tasks of prevention as well as care, affected communities are not enabled to become involved. The full engagement of affected communities and those who are potentially affected in the MENA/EM region requires a renewed effort at working with NGOs. Laws that limit their access to resources or other activities may need review and change. NGOs must be invited to join governments and other actors in a renewed effort to maintain low prevalence where it really exists and reduce the number of new cases where prevalence is higher, as in Djibouti.

Empowering local communities, through NGOs or similar agencies, requires a process of rapprochement and a reversal in some respects of the current top-down approach to HIV prevention. Action research conducted with vulnerable groups can heighten the groups' own awareness of the potential threat to themselves from HIV and galvanize their interest in responding. NGO ombudsmen could serve to facilitate ongoing dialogue between governments and NGOs.

Monitoring and Evaluation

National programs have formally evaluated their progress in only a few cases. All have reported to WHO/EMRO at intercountry meetings, but these reports often gloss over the gaps and difficulties encountered.

Proper monitoring and evaluation of the investments made require adequate second-generation surveillance as well as independent teams brought in to evaluate the programs periodically. This is a critical mechanism to bring about continued improvement.

The Time Required

Successfully implementing the programs described above, including improved second-generation surveillance, takes a considerable amount of time. While the needed technical expertise to carry out these activities may not be found in each country, it can be found in the region or in other similar cultural environments.

A regional network of experts on HIV/AIDS could be facilitated by UNAIDS. Building up local capacity should always be a high priority, but it requires many years of investment.

Behavior change also requires time. Many people are unable to change their risky behaviors without considerable support. This situation has to be understood, and appropriate services must be developed.

Financing the Effort

When political commitment is evident, funds are more likely to be found. The World Bank is an appropriate source for government-led major programs. Bilateral donors more often can give directly to NGOs and fund specific, time-limited projects. The GFATM is a new and valuable source of funding. Sustainability, however, must be considered. Ultimately, people need to learn how to protect their own sexual/reproductive health or to seek treatment for their addictions. The products and services required must be available, even if these are eventually purchased. A long-term plan to incorporate specific services into national insurance schemes or other health plans should be considered. None of these actions will be acceptable unless the public understands what HIV and STDs are, how they affect health, and how they can avoid these diseases. Improved sexual/reproductive health services for both men and women as well as improved drug-dependence treatment may require a fee-for-service approach. This approach would not only ensure greater

financial sustainability but, in the best of circumstances, would also subject these services to consumer pressure and make them adjust to consumer needs and preferences.

In the short term, the government of each country in the MENA/EM
region must begin to consider HIV a national issue of great importance,
with the potential to produce damaging and costly consequences for the
nation. In the long term, such services should be mainstreamed into the
regular health and social welfare services and public health disease-pre-
vention activities.

Immediate Next Steps

Recommendations for improving the current situation include:

- Raising the priority given to HIV/AIDS through research, media, and
  advocacy.

- Evaluating what national HIV/AIDS/STD programs have achieved,
  including proposing ways to strengthen them.

- Developing national policy and strategic plans, with associated budgets and the identification of potential resources.

- Instituting second-generation surveillance, including STD and behavioral surveys.

- Learning to conduct targeted interventions with at-risk groups in a
  quiet, culturally appropriate manner, in collaboration with NGOs.

- Reducing the vulnerability of migrants, internally displaced persons
  (IDP), mobile populations, and refugees with the involvement of
  U.N. agencies and appropriate INGOs, beginning with research to
  assess situations of risk followed by a process involving all stakeholders to design appropriate and coordinated interventions.

- Improving the provision of clear information and means of protection, and taking small steps toward the development of adequate promotion of condoms.

- Developing life skills and drug demand–reduction education for
  youth that is culturally appropriate and effective and recognizes the
  structural factors associated with drug use.

- Reducing vulnerability among youth through multisectoral planning
  to affect sexual and reproductive health, unemployment rates, educational costs, and information access, among other critical issues.

- Ensuring that ART programs are provided and include adequate prevention services as well.

- Empowering affected communities by encouraging local NGO development, including increased participation of PLWHA.

- Developing regional networks of experts to fulfill technical needs while developing local capacity.

- Developing programs based on sound knowledge of situational context, with increased participation from a wide range of sectors and partners, which addresses vulnerability factors and includes monitoring and evaluation plans and budgets.

- Considering future sustainability through insurance and other health financing schemes that can help ensure equitable access to health care for people of all socioeconomic strata.

- Strengthening country-level information systems, in order to monitor and evaluate the situation and response to HIV/AIDS.

- Mobilizing additional human and financial resources in support of national responses through collaborative efforts involving a wider range of international, regional, and national partnerships.

These actions require the collaborative effort of many agencies across the U.N. system, multiple sectors within government, CBOs, INGOs, bilateral donors, and religious and other local leaders. Most of all, the coordination of such a program requires political commitment at the highest level. If that commitment is attained, the MENA/EM region can avert the threat that HIV represents to its development goals. The time to act is today, when prevalence is still low.

Technical Appendix

Exploring the Socioeconomic Determinants of HIV/AIDS Prevalence Levels

This book uses the results of two cross-country studies: a first study conducted by Over (1997) and a second study conducted by the authors of this paper. The methodology in both cases is similar. The differences reside in the type of variables and countries included in the analysis. Over's study uses subnational data and focuses on urban HIV/AIDS prevalence levels. Our study uses national data and focuses on aggregate prevalence levels.

The statistical models estimated are of the form:

$$\log\left(\frac{h_i}{H - h_i}\right) = \mathbf{X}_i\beta + \mu_i \; ; i \in \mathbf{I} \tag{1}$$

where h is the HIV prevalence level, H is the maximum prevalence level that can be observed, X is a vector of explanatory variables, β is a vector of parameters to be estimated, m are random shocks, and I is the set of countries. The two studies differ in terms of the variables included in X as well as the countries included in I. Both studies estimate model (1) using ordinary least squares. Endogeneity problems are addressed by including lagged variables in X. For instance, in the case of our analysis, HIV prevalence levels (h) correspond to 1999, while the socioeconomic indicators correspond to 1997.

Table A.1 summarizes the results from Over (1997). Tables A.2 and A.3 present the estimates of the current study. The difference between tables A.2 and A.3 is the inclusion/exclusion of the *female labor force participation rate* as an explanatory variable. The first column of each table describes the explanatory variables (the Xs), the second column contains estimates for the coefficients (the βs), and the third column gives the ratio between the coefficient and its standard deviation. Ratios above 1.6 indicate that the coefficient has at least a 90 percent probability of being different from zero.

TABLE A.1

Estimates of Model 1

Observations	132		
Prob > F	0		
R-squared	0.621		
Variable		Coefficient	t-Statistic
Age of epidemic		0.63	5.5
GNP per capita (log)		−1.2	−5.2
Foreign-born percentage of the population		0.25	1.9
Percentage of Muslims		−0.013	−3.2
Gini index of inequality		7.9	3.7
Male-female literacy gap		0.051	2.2
Urban male/female gender ratio, ages 20–39		2.4	1.9
Military forces as a percentage of the urban population		0.056	3.1
Constant		−8.5	−2.7

Note: 132 observations correspond to 72 countries. GNP, gross national product.
Source: Over 1997.

TABLE A.2

Estimates of Model 2, Excluding Female Participation in the Labor Force

Observations	93			
Prob > F	0			
R-squared	0.7044			

Variable	Coefficient	Standard error	t	Probability coefficient is different from zero (percent)
GDP per capita (log)	3.457995	1.05874	3.29	99.80
Gini coefficient	0.043984	0.02449	1.8	92.40
Female illiteracy (log)	−0.47499	0.210863	−2.25	97.30
Indicator for Africa	38.31385	10.88467	3.52	99.90
Indicator for Asia	37.15606	10.35637	3.59	99.90
Indicator for Eastern Europe and Central Asia	33.21808	10.83085	3.07	99.70
Indicator for Latin America	33.96994	10.51811	3.23	99.80
Indicator for the Middle East and North Africa	30.93839	9.345694	3.31	99.90
GDP per capita effect in Africa	−3.62468	1.289511	−2.81	99.40
GDP per capita effect in Asia	−3.94852	1.135634	−3.48	99.90
GDP per capita effect in Europe and Central Asia	−3.69679	1.176082	−3.14	99.80
GDP per capita effect in Latin American and the Caribbean	−3.46205	1.166691	−2.97	99.60
GDP per capita effect in the Middle East and North Africa	−3.35197	1.015941	−3.3	99.90
Constant	−39.0636	10.267	−3.8	100.00

Note: GDP, gross domestic product.
Source: Authors' calculations.

TABLE A.3

Estimates of Model 2, Including Female Participation in the Labor Force

Observations	91
Prob > F	0
R-squared	0.7109

Variable	Coefficient	Standard error	t	Probability coefficient is different from zero (percent)
GDP per capita (log)	3.511863	0.99	3.54	99.90
Gini coefficient	0.0429746	0.02	1.78	92.10
Share of females in the labor force (square)	−46.83818	30.43	−1.54	87.20
Share of females in the labor force (log squared)	6.750899	4.29	1.57	88.00
Female illiteracy (log)	−0.3944203	0.23	−1.69	90.40
Indicator for Africa	36.09592	10.14	3.56	99.90
Indicator for Asia	35.70654	9.66	3.7	100.00
Indicator for Eastern Europe and Central Asia	31.3269	10.33	3.03	99.70
Indicator for Latin America	35.099	9.68	3.62	99.90
Indicator for the Middle East and North Africa	31.38874	8.89	3.53	99.90
GDP per capita effect in Africa	−3.384934	1.20	−2.81	99.40
GDP per capita effect in Asia	−3.802523	1.06	−3.58	99.90
GDP per capita effect in Europe and Central Asia	−3.546957	1.12	−3.16	99.80
GDP per capita effect in Latin America and the Caribbean	−3.581975	1.07	−3.36	99.90
GDP per capita effect in the Middle East and North Africa	−3.41716	0.96	−3.54	99.90
Constant	41.30813	53.60	0.77	55.70

Note: GDP, gross domestic product.
Source: Author's calculations.

Estimating the Potential Socioeconomic Impacts of the Epidemic

Our model focuses on four channels through which the epidemic affects the economy: the size and composition of the labor force, productivity growth, health expenditures, and the savings rate of the economy. Other channels, such as reductions in human capital resulting from an increase in the number of orphans, who are less likely to fully develop their physical and intellectual capacities,[1] are ignored for methodological reasons. Thus, it can be said that our model underestimates the economic cost of the HIV/AIDS epidemic.

The model has been modified from its original version (Robalino, Voetberg, and Picaso 2002) in two important ways. First, we introduce three types of labor that can be affected differently by the epidemic: skilled labor, unskilled labor, and unemployed labor. Second, we couple the macroeconomic model to an HIV/AIDS diffusion model that simultaneously takes into account sexual transmission and transmission through the sharing of infected needles among IDUs (the two major transmission mechanisms in the case of MENA/EM countries). This is a convenient feature of the model because it allows us to simulate the welfare implications of specific interventions such as increasing condom use and access to clean needles for IDUs.

Another important feature of the model is that the savings rate of the economy is computed endogenously to maximize intertemporal consumption. This allows us to simulate the impacts of the epidemics under "ideal conditions" and to take a normative stance in terms of when and how governments should intervene.[2] In fact, the assumption introduced in most models that savings are reduced as a result of the epidemics is not supported by empirical data. In the absence of well-functioning insurance markets, rational agents may actually increase savings to protect themselves against potentially high future health expenditures. The ultimate effect that HIV/AIDS has on the savings rate of the economy will depend on how it affects agents' preferences (risk aversion, discount rates) and governments' fiscal balance. For simplicity, our simulations will keep preferences constant and assume that societies respond optimally to the shock resulting from the epidemics. This could underestimate the macroeconomic impacts of the epidemic.

Modeling the Economy

The model is based on the assumption that the output of a given economy can be represented as a simple function of labor and capital:

$$Y_t = H^{1-\theta} K_t^{\theta} A_t \tag{1}$$

where Y is GDP, K is the stock of produced capital, H is quality-adjusted labor, our proxy for human capital, and A is a scale factor.

The growth rate of A captures changes in total factor productivity, and its dynamics are determined exogenously. Thus, we have:

$$\log A_t = \log A_{t-1} + \gamma_a \exp(-\delta_a t) \tag{2}$$

where γ_a is the growth rate of aggregate labor productivity and δ_a is the yearly reduction in this growth rate.

Human capital is defined by:

$$H_t = \sum_i a_i N_{it}; \quad i \in I \tag{3}$$

where N_i is the number of workers of type i, a_i is the productivity of labor type i, and I is the set of labor types. It is convenient to rewrite equation (3) as:

$$H_t = q_t N_t \qquad (4)$$

where q_t is the average quality of labor at time t, given by:

$$q_t = \frac{1}{N_t} \sum_i a_i N_{it}; \quad i \in \mathbf{I} \qquad (5)$$

For simplicity in this application, we use three types of labor: skilled ($a = 1$), unskilled (arbitrarily defined by $a = 0.5$), and unemployed ($a = 0$). Given little knowledge about the operation of the labor markets in the MENA/EM region, we have avoided modeling explicitly its dynamics (by formalizing labor supply and demand decisions). Instead, we make assumptions about transition probabilities between different types of labor and treat the growth rate of the aggregate labor force exogenously. This treatment is sufficient to achieve our objective of being able to simulate the impact of alternative distributions of the burden of HIV/AIDS across the labor force. Thus, we postulate:

$$\mathbf{N}_t = \eta_1 \left[\mathbf{N}_{t-1} - \mathbf{D}_{t-1} \right] + \eta_2' \Delta N_t \qquad (6)$$

where N is a (3,1) vector giving the number of workers in each labor class, η_1 is a (3,3) matrix of transition probabilities, D is a (3,1) vector giving the number of deaths in each labor class, η_2 is a (1,3) vector giving the share of new workers going to each labor class, and ΔN is the number of new workers.

This number of new workers is characterized as follows:

$$\begin{cases} N_t = \exp\left[\log(N_{t-1}) + \gamma_n \exp(-\delta_n t)\right] - \Delta H_{t-10} \\ H_t = \beta_t N_t \end{cases} \qquad (7)$$

where H is the total number of HIV/AIDS-infected individuals and β is the aggregate HIV/AIDS prevalence level. This function underestimates the demographic impact of the epidemic. We use it for analytical simplicity.

To derive the optimal savings rate, and therefore the dynamics of the stock of produced capital, we assume that economies will operate along a path that maximizes a utility function that depends on aggregate consumption. More specifically, we solve the following optimization problem:

$$\text{Max}_c: V(C_t) = \sum_t \rho^t \left\{ N_t \frac{(C_t/N_t)^\tau}{1-\tau} \right\}$$

$$\text{s.t.:,} \quad K_t = K_{t-1}(1-\delta_k) + (Y_t - C_t) \tag{8}$$

$$(1), (2), (4), \text{ and } (5)$$

where δ_k is the depreciation of capital, ρ is a discount factor, and τ is the coefficient of risk aversion. We use a standard constant elasticity of substitution value function that is population weighted. By aggregating across the population, we are able to capture part of the welfare losses resulting from premature deaths.[3]

It can be shown that under optimal conditions, the dynamics of the stock of produced capital can be approximated by:

$$\Delta \ln \left(K_{t+1}/N_{t+1} \right) = \alpha_1 + \alpha_2 \left(\ln \left(K_{t+1}/N_{t+1} \right) - \ln(T_t) \right) \tag{9}$$

where $T_1 = q_1 A_t^{1/(1-\theta)}$, and α_1 and α_2 are functions of the sequence $\{q_t\}$, the growth rate of the labor force, and of the parameters γ_a, δ_k, θ, τ, and ρ (see Robalino, Voetberg, and Picaso 2002).

Up to here, in this model, the HIV/AIDS epidemic affects the size of the labor force and its composition, thus affecting the dynamics of the quality of the labor force and the savings rate of the economy (through equation 9). We also consider the possibility that, for a given composition of the labor force, the HIV/AIDS prevalence level affects the aggregate level of productivity. As discussed previously, this may occur as labor turnover and absenteeism increase and as firms divert resources to preventive activities. This can also occur if economic efficiency decreases as resources are allocated to treat HIV/AIDS patients. To formalize this idea, we simply postulate that the realized level of productivity is given by:

$$A_t^* = A_t \left(1 - d_1 \beta_t - d_2 c_{ht} \right) \tag{10}$$

where d_1 and d_2 are the parameters determining productivity losses, and c_h is the share of HIV/AIDS health-related expenditures in GDP. In the presence of HIV/AIDS, A^* replaces A in equations (1) to (9).

Health expenditures are simply modeled by keeping track of an average expenditure per patient (which depends on the level of GDP per capita) and a given level of access to health services. We have:

$$c_{h,t} = \left(\lambda_0 (y_t)^{\lambda_1} \lambda_2 H_t \right) / Y_t \tag{11}$$

where λ_0 and λ_1 are the parameters determining the average cost of treating an HIV/AIDS patient as a function of GDP per capita (y), and λ_2 gives the share of the stock H of infected individuals who have access to curative services.

Modeling the Diffusion of HIV/AIDS

As with any other infectious disease, the diffusion of HIV/AIDS depends on its reproduction rate. This is the average number of people who are infected by a person carrying the virus during his or her life span. The higher the reproduction rate, the faster the diffusion of the disease. Diseases that have a reproduction rate lower than 1 gradually disappear. In the case of HIV/AIDS, the reproduction rate is determined by the types of contagion mechanisms (sexual intercourse, sharing of infected needles among drug users, mother to child, blood transfusion, or repeated use of needles in hospitals and health centers), and three elements associated with each of them: (a) the duration of the period during which an individual can transmit the disease through the given mechanism, (b) the risk of transmission per contact, and (c) the frequency and heterogeneity of contacts. In this study, the focus is on sexual transmission and transmission through the sharing of infected needles among drug users. These are the main channels through which the epidemic can diffuse in MENA/EM countries.[4] Research has also shown that it is very unlikely that HIV/AIDS could have a sustainable diffusion rate if the only transmission mechanisms were mother to child, blood transfusions, or the repeated use of needles in hospitals and health centers.

Duration of the Infecting Period

The absence of a treatment to cure the disease and long survival periods characterize HIV. Thus, unlike other diseases, HIV has a long period during which the disease can be transmitted, and this length of time increases its reproduction rate. The fact that the disease can be asymptomatic for several years also contributes to a high reproduction rate. Since little can be done to reduce the infecting period from a medical point of view, it is usually treated as a constant in epidemiological models (that is, the infecting period is not affected by changes in the economic and social environments).

Risk of Transmission per Contact

In the case of unprotected sexual intercourse, the probability of transmission of HIV/AIDS is relatively low when compared with other

STDs. In industrial countries, for instance, the probability of transmission from an infected man to a woman is approximately 0.1 percent to 0.2 percent, while the probability of transmission from an infected woman to a man is half of that. Nonetheless, these numbers could underestimate transmission probabilities in developing countries, where sanitary conditions are poorer than in industrial countries (for example, the prevalence of STDs that contribute to the transmission of HIV is higher).[5] In the case of infected needles, the probability of contagion is greater (in the order of 3 per 100 contacts) than in the case of unprotected sexual contacts, although it varies with the type of materials used and how the drug is administered. In general, this mechanism contributes to a high reproduction rate, because the epidemic can diffuse to the majority of the population of drug users within a few months (see table A.6 for assumptions about transmission probabilities).

Frequency and Heterogeneity of Exchanges

The frequency of exchanges of sexual or drug partners is likely to be the main factor determining diffusion patterns. Other things being equal, the higher the frequency of exchange, the higher the reproduction rate. The heterogeneity of these exchanges also plays a key role. Indeed, if exchanges are limited to a population with similar sexual or drug-use patterns, say a high-risk population group in which individuals change partners frequently, the epidemic would fail to diffuse to the remaining low-risk part of the population. Thus, in theory, the epidemic could be localized to specific risk groups, and although the aggregate prevalence level can initially increase rapidly, it would usually stabilize at low levels, as individuals of the high-risk group die. In practice, however, this is rarely the case. The most common situation is when interactions are heterogeneous in the sense that there are interactions between low-risk and high-risk groups. In this case, the epidemic can rapidly progress to the entire population. Individuals' behaviors and the distribution of the epidemic among different risk groups therefore play a key role in determining diffusion patterns.

Our model simulates the spread of HIV/AIDS through two channels: sharing of infected needles among IDUs and sexual intercourse. The former is based on Law (2001), while the latter is based on the AVERT model developed in Rehle and others (1998). AVERT was modified to consider additional population groups (the original model has only two population groups) and to introduce time (the original model is static).[6]

The model divides a country's population aged 15 to 49 years into five groups: prostitutes, female IDUs, male IDUs, low-risk females, and low-risk males. In terms of infections related to needle sharing, the model assumes that needles are shared at random (this assumption is introduced for tractability). Hence, the probability that an uninfected IDU would become infected between time t – 1 and t is given by:

$$\Pr_{it} = 1 - \left\{ \sum_d \phi_d \left[\beta_{dt} \left(1 - r_{idu} \right) + \left(1 - \beta_d \right) \right] \right\}^{n(1-u-dU)} \qquad i \in D \quad \forall \quad d \in \{(12)$$

where D is the vector of IDU population groups (in this case, D has two elements: male and female), ϕ_d is the share of the population of group d in the total population of IDUs, β_{dt} is the HIV/AIDS prevalence in the population group d, r_{idu} is the probability of infection after an injection with an infected needle, n is the total number of injections between time t – 1 and time t, u is the share of these injections that use safe needles, and dU is a policy variable introduced to simulate reductions in sharing practices. In equation (12), the expression between { } is the probability of remaining uninfected after an injection with a shared needle. The probability that the needle will come from group d is given by ϕ_d. Within this group, the probability that the needle is infected is given by β_d, the HIV/AIDS prevalence level in group d. Finally, if the needle is infected, the probability that the individual will not acquire HIV is given by 1 – r_{idu}. To obtain the joint probability of remaining uninfected after n injections, taking into account that a share $1 - u - dU$ of these injections takes place through shared needles, we simply raise the expression in brackets to the n $(1 - u - dU)$ power.

In the simulations, before considering infections resulting from sexual intercourse, the prevalence level for the IDUs population groups is updated on the basis of equation (12). We get:

$$\beta_{dt} = \left(H_{dt} + N_{dt} \left(1 - \beta_{dt} \right) \Pr_{dt} \right) / N_{dt} \qquad (13)$$

where H_{dt} is the stock of HIV/AIDS-infected individuals at time t in group d. At this stage, deaths are not yet taken into account.

In terms of infections transmitted sexually, we follow the same mechanics as the model AVERT. The probability that an HIV-negative individual would become infected at time t is given by:

$$\Pr_{it} = 1 - \prod_j \left\{ \left[\beta_{jt} \left(\sum_s w_s \left(1 - r_s \left(1 - \left(f + dF \right) e \right) \right) \right)^{n_{ij}} + \left(1 - \beta_{jt} \right) \right]^{m_{ij}} \right\} \qquad (14)$$

$$i \in J; j \in J_{-i}; s \in S$$

where J is the vector of population groups (five, in this case), β_{jt} is the HIV/AIDS prevalence observed in group j at time t, S is a vector containing different STDs status (four cases are considered: non-STDs, ulcerative STDs, nonulcerative STDs, and both ulcerative and nonulcerative), w_s is the probability of observing state s, r_s is the probability of HID/AIDS transmission after intercourse in status s, f is the probability of using condoms, e is the effectiveness of the condoms, m_{ij} is the average number of sexual partners that individuals of group i have in group j, and n_{ij} is the average number of intercourses with each partner between time t and t + 1. Similar to the case of equation (12), the expression between { } gives the probability that an uninfected individual in group i would remain uninfected after sexual intercourse with m_{ij} partners in group j. The product over the J groups gives the joint probability of remaining uninfected after sexual intercourse with the partners in all groups. Inside the brackets, the probability that the partner will be infected with HIV is approximated by the prevalence level β_j. If the partner is infected, the probability of remaining uninfected after n_{ij} intercourses is given by the expression in parentheses. The probability of infection is given by r_s, which depends on whether the partner suffers from an STD. The probability of having different types of STDs is given by w_s. Therefore, the sum gives the expected probability of remaining uninfected after one intercourse with a partner, taking into account the prevalence of STDs.

Under these assumptions, the dynamics of the HIV/AIDS prevalence level is given by:

$$\beta_{t+1} = \left(\sum_j \left(H_{jt} + N_{jt}\left(1-\beta_{jt}\right)\mathrm{Pr}_{jt} - \Delta H_{jt-10} \right) \right) / N_{t+1} \qquad (15)$$

Model Calibration

The different model parameters are summarized in tables A.4 to A.6. Table A.4 is divided into four sections. The first section defines economic parameters (those determining growth and the dynamics of labor markets). The third section defines parameters determining the economic impact of the epidemic for a given prevalence level. Finally, the fourth section concerns the parameters affecting the diffusion of the epidemic. Tables A.5 and A.6 present additional parameters affecting this diffusion. We discuss each of these in turn.

Economic Parameters

Economic parameters are grouped into two categories: *growth parameters* and *labor market* parameters. Among the 10 growth parameters, three were defined exogenously and are fixed across countries: the depreciation rate of capital (d_k), the discount rate (r), and the coefficient of risk aversion in the utility function (t). The other parameters along with one of the labor market parameters (the share of unemployed workers who find a job) were estimated in order to achieve targets in terms of medium- and long-term economic growth, investment targets, and demographic projections. We proceeded as follows. The growth rate of the labor force (g_N) and the change in the growth rate of the labor force (d_N) were estimated on the basis of the World Bank official country projections. The remaining parameters, the labor productivity growth (l_A), the change in the growth rate of labor productivity growth (d_A), the coefficient of the labor factor in the production function (q), and the share of unemployed workers who find a job (h_{13}) were estimated by solving the following optimization problem:

$$
Min_{\gamma_a, \delta_a, \theta, \eta_{13}} : \left[g(1-5) - \left(Y_5 / Y_1 \right)^{1/4} \right]^2 +
$$

$$
\left[g(5-15) - \left(Y_{15} / Y_5 \right)^{1/10} \right]^2 +
$$

$$
\left[g(15-25) - \left(Y_{25} / Y_{15} \right)^{1/20} \right]^2 +
$$

$$
\left[I(1-25) - \frac{1}{25} \sum_{t=1}^{t=25} s_t \right]^2
$$

where $g(t-z)$ represents targets for the average growth rate during year t and year z, and $I(t-z)$ gives targets for the average saving rate during the period $t - z$. These targets were set for each country on the basis of the Country Assistance Strategies (World Bank 1997a, 1997b, 1999b, 1999c, 2000c, 2001b, 2001c, 2001d; World Bank Group 2001). Long-term growth rates increase the medium-term targets by 1 percent. Investment rates are based on the average of the past 10 years. When this average is below 20 percent, 20 percent is used instead.

In terms of labor market parameters, initial unemployment rates come from World Bank Country Assistance Strategies (World Bank 1997a, 1997b, 1999b, 1999c, 2000c, 2001b, 2001c, 2001d; World Bank Group

TABLE A.4

Model Parameters

	Algeria	Djibouti	Egypt, Arab Rep. of	Iran, Islamic Rep. of	Jordan	Lebanon	Morocco	Tunisia	Yemen, Rep. of
Economic parameters									
Growth parameters	3.717099109	4.4721018	3.340365209	3.190799434	4.79784352	3	4.385460769	3.082643516	2.306631591
deltaK	0.04000	0.04000	0.04000	0.04000	0.04000	0.04000	0.04000	0.04000	0.04000
deltaA	0.00500	0.00500	0.00500	0.00500	0.00500	0.00500	0.00500	0.00500	0.01000
deltaN	0.05200	0.01416	0.03627	0.07246	0.04181	0.11327	0.05036	0.08827	0.01323
lambdaA	0.03690	0.00386	0.04017	0.01937	0.01360	0.02734	0.02617	0.05357	0.00100
lambdaN	0.03162	0.02396	0.02350	0.03538	0.03951	0.03575	0.02220	0.02705	0.03868
rho	0.06000	0.06000	0.06000	0.06000	0.06000	0.06000	0.06000	0.06000	0.06000
tau	0.90000	0.90000	0.90000	0.90000	0.90000	0.90000	0.90000	0.90000	0.90000
theta	0.48337	0.24010	0.33260	0.27609	0.32662	0.34267	0.36577	0.42584	0.20954
alfa1	0.31056	0.23486	0.18673	0.15346	0.16536	0.26148	0.23544	0.47009	0.43993
alfa2	-0.14861	-0.11626	-0.07217	-0.08636	-0.06166	-0.16948	-0.08978	-0.28734	-0.40277
Labor markets									
Share unemployed	21%	40%	11%	15%	10%	15%	20%	15%	30%
Share skilled labor	50%	50%	50%	50%	50%	50%	50%	50%	50%
Share unemployed in new labor	0%	0%	0%	0%	0%	0%	0%	0%	0%
Share skilled in new labor	70%	70%	70%	70%	70%	70%	70%	70%	70%
Share unemployed who find a job	1.27%	0.13%	1.46%	0.38%	0.40%	0.53%	0.58%	0.99%	0.01%
Constraints									
s(2001–10)	0.27827	0.20000	0.24458	0.20000	0.25000	0.20500	0.25000	0.27849	0.20000
g(2000–05)	0.04525	0.03475	0.05500	0.03767	0.04000	0.03600	0.04000	0.05700	0.04000
g(2005–15)	0.05025	0.03975	0.06000	0.04267	0.04500	0.04100	0.04500	0.06200	0.04500
Initial conditions (million GDP 1995)	0.00000	0.00000	0.00000	0.00000	0.00000	0.00000	0.00000	0.00000	0.00000
COR*	5.03310	2.00000	2.69900	2.67200	3.20300	3.50000	3.16900	3.62600	2.00000
Y	47,085.0	486.0	74,610.0	99,920.4	7,604.0	12,358.6	38,387.0	22,600.0	4,880.0
C	34,123.4	440.3	57,607.4	81,708.9	6,023.6	9,639.7	29,110.6	16,583.6	3,972.6
I/Y	0.3	0.1	0.2	0.2	0.2	0.2	0.2	0.3	0.2

K	175,019.6	2,173.4	249,224.6	318,825.9	36,482.8	37,075.8	168,344.7	69,667.7	11,256.4
A	0.0	0.0	0.0	0.0	0.0	0.0	0.0	0.0	0.0
N	16.0	0.3	34.3	34.4	3.1	1.7	15.1	5.2	7.6
Impacts of the epidemic									
Share AIDS–related deceased among skilled	[20%–50%]	[20%–50%]	[20%–50%]	[20%–50%]	[20%–50%]	[20%–50%]	[20%–50%]	[20%–50%]	[20%–50%]
Impact labor productivity (d1)	[0–1]	[0–1]	[0–1]	[0–1]	[0–1]	[0–1]	[0–1]	[0–1]	[0–1]
Impact health spending (d2)	0	0	0	0	0	0	0	0	0
Initial cost of AIDS treatment/GDP	1.5	1.5	1.5	1.5	1.5	1.5	1.5	1.5	1.5
Marginal increase in the cost	0.95	0.95	0.95	0.95	0.95	0.95	0.95	0.95	0.95
Access to treatment	0.3	0.3	0.3	0.3	0.3	0.3	0.3	0.3	0.3
HIV/AIDS diffusion									
Epidemiology									
Baseline share sex workers + [0%–0.5%]	0.31%	1.00%	0.31%	0.31%	0.31%	0.31%	0.31%	0.31%	0.30%
Baseline share IDUs1 + [0%–0.5%]	0.05%	0.00%	0.05%	0.05%	0.00%	0.05%	0.05%	0.05%	0.00%
Baseline share IDUs2 + [0%–0.5%]	0.05%	0.00%	0.05%	0.05%	0.00%	0.05%	0.05%	0.05%	0.00%
Share infected sex workers + [0%–5%]	10.00%	15.00%	1.00%	1.00%	1.00%	1.00%	1.00%	1.00%	7.00%
Share infected IDUs1 + [0%–5%]	0.30%	0.00%	1.00%	1.00%	0.00%	2.20%	0.34%	0.34%	0.00%
Share infected IDUs2 + [0%–5%]	0.30%	0.00%	1.00%	1.00%	0.00%	2.20%	0.34%	0.34%	0.00%
Aggregate prevalence rate	0.07%	3.00%	0.02%	0.03%	0.02%	0.09%	0.03%	0.06%	0.02%
Preventive/health behavior									
Condom use	[10%–50%]	[10%–50%]	[10%–50%]	[10%–50%]	[10%–50%]	[10%–50%]	[10%–50%]	[10%–50%]	[10%–50%]
Condom effectiveness	98.00%	98.00%	98.00%	98.00%	98.00%	98.00%	98.00%	98.00%	98.00%
Needle sharing	[10%–50%]	[10%–50%]	[10%–50%]	[10%–50%]	[10%–50%]	[10%–50%]	[10%–50%]	[10%–50%]	[10%–50%]
Average number of injections per year	730	730	730	730	730	730	730	730	
STD prevalence	[0%–5%]	[0%–5%]	[0%–5%]	[0%–5%]	[0%–5%]	[0%–5%]	[0%–5%]	[0%–5%]	[0%–5%]

Note: A, total factor productivity; C, consumption; COR, capital output ratio; GDP, gross domestic product; IDU, injecting drug user; I/Y, share of investment in GDP; K, capital; N, labor; STD, sexually transmitted disease; Y, GDP.

Source: Authors' calculations.

2001). For simplicity, the initial share of skilled workers is arbitrarily set equal to 50 percent and kept fixed across countries. The share of unskilled laborers is then computed by difference. We take an optimistic stance, assuming that new entrants in the labor force are not unemployed and that a majority, 70 percent, are skilled. We do not allow mobility across labor types (except from the unemployed group to the skilled).

The initial conditions for the output variables are set on the basis of the World Bank SIMA (World Bank 2002b) and, in the case of the capital output ratio, using the World Bank Total Factor Productivity tool kit. We note that all the economic parameters are fixed across simulations.

Parameters Affecting the Impact of the Epidemic

Three sets of parameters determine the economic impact of the epidemic: (a) the parameters affecting the distribution of HIV/AIDS-related deaths among labor types, (b) the parameters determining HIV/AIDS-related health expenditures and the impact on productivity, and (c) the parameter determining the direct impact of the HIV/AIDS prevalence rate on labor productivity.

In terms of the distribution of AIDS-related deaths, given little or no data in that respect, we allow the share of skilled workers to vary between 20 percent and 50 percent. The higher this share, the larger the economic impacts. By considering a maximum value of 50 percent, we take a conservative approach. The remaining deaths are equally distributed among low-skilled and unemployed workers.

The calculation of potential changes in health expenditures is based on estimates from the literature. In terms of the average cost of treatment, estimates from cross-country studies suggest a range of two to three times GDP per capita (Cyrillo, Paulani, and Aguirre 2001; Floyd and Gilks 2001). In this analysis, we assume that the average yearly cost of treating an HIV/AIDS patient is equal to US$1,400 in a country with a GDP per capita of US$1,000 and that it increases by 0.95 percent for each 1 percent increase in GDP per capita. Access to treatment, however, varies widely across countries. For our calculations, we assume that only a modest 30 percent of those affected by AIDS would obtain treatment. For simplicity, we neglect the effects that higher health expenditures may have on productivity growth.

Finally, the parameter defining the direct impact of HIV/AIDS on labor productivity is allowed to vary between 0 and 0.5. This implies that a 1 percent prevalence level can reduce the growth rate of labor productivity by up to 0.5 percentage point from its baseline. This is the low range from estimates in the literature (Haacker 2001; MacFarlan and Sgherri 2001).

Parameters Determining the Diffusion of the Epidemic

Given the lack of epidemiological and behavioral data, we allow the different parameters to vary uniformly along wide intervals. We start by defining the approximate HIV/AIDS prevalence level in the general population and prevalence levels among high-risk groups (sex workers and IDUs). For this, we use UNAIDS country profiles and data collected for this study. In the case of Morocco, where data on the prevalence level of IDUs are not available, we assume levels equivalent to Tunisia. There are no reliable data regarding the population share of sex workers and IDUs in the different countries. Thus, we treat these shares as exogenous parameters that are allowed to change between simulations from a conservative baseline; changes range between 0 percent and 0.5 percent. Given the share of the different population groups, the aggregate prevalence level, and the prevalence levels for the high-risk groups (which are also allowed to vary between 0 percent and 0.5 percent), we compute the implicit prevalence levels for the low-risk groups. There are also scarce data regarding sex behaviors and drug use. The probability of using a condom is allowed to vary between 10 percent (close to Morocco) and 50 percent (close to Jordan). The probability of sharing a needle is allowed to vary between 10 percent and 50 percent, while the average number of injections per year is fixed at 730 (see Jenkins, Rahman, and others 2001). Finally, the STD prevalence is allowed to vary between 0 percent and 5 percent. The total number of STD cases is equally divided among nonulcerative, ulcerative, and both.

The second important set of parameters that affects the dynamics of the HIV/AIDS epidemic is given by the level and heterogeneity of sexual activity. Table A.5 presents the average number of partners across population groups and the average number of occurrences of intercourse. The numbers are based on Rehle and others (1998). Given high uncertainty about the correct values across countries, we also allow these parameters to vary (all in the same proportion). The matrices are thus multiplied in different simulations by a scalar ranging between 0.5 and 2.

The final set of model parameters relates to HIV/AIDS transmission probabilities. In the case of sexual transmission, we allow the probability of infection to vary as a function of the presence of the three different types of STDs (ulcerative, nonulcerative, and both). The different probabilities are summarized in table A.6.

(*Text continues on page 125.*)

Average Number of Partners and of Occurrences of Intercourse per Year

	Sex workers	Male IDUs	Female IDUs	Low-risk males	Low-risk females
Partners					
Sex workers	0	5	0	15	0
Male IDUs	32	0	2	0	1
Female IDUs	0	2	0	2	0
Low-risk males	0.0932	0	0.0019	0	2
Low-risk females	0	0.0010	0	2	0
	Sex workers	Male IDUs	Female IDUs	Low-risk males	Low-risk females
Contacts					
Sex workers	0	7	0	7	0
Male IDUs	7	0	7	0	7
Female IDUs	0	7	0	7	0
Low-risk males	7	0	7	0	25
Low-risk females	0	7	0	25	0

Note: IDU, injecting drug user.
Source: Based on Rehle and others 1998.

HIV/AIDS Transmission Probabilities

	No STD	Ulcerative STD	Nonulcerative STD	Ulcerative and nonulcerative STD	Infected needle
Probability of transmission	0.002	0.04	0.02	0.04	0.03

Note: STD, sexually transmitted disease.
Source: Rehle and others 1998.

Summary of the Results of the Simulations

TABLE A.7

Descriptive Statistics for Output Variables: Status Quo

Country	Statistic	pvGDP [2000–25] loss (percentage of today's GDP)	Average GDP growth rate, 2000–25 (percent)	Population change in 2025, (percent)	HIV prevalence, 2015 (percent)	Health expenditures, 2015 (percentage of GDP)
Algeria	Mean	41.2	−0.40	−4.1	4.5	1.5
	Standard deviation	53.0	0.63	4.9	6.4	2.2
	Minimum	2.8	−4.36	−35.0	0.1	0.0
	Maximum	363.9	−0.01	−0.3	45.4	15.4
Djibouti	Mean	150.8	−1.34	−16.7	15.9	5.6
	Standard deviation	114.8	1.43	13.1	16.4	5.8
	Minimum	31.6	−7.02	−69.3	0.6	0.2
	Maximum	609.4	−0.15	−3.6	79.2	28.4
Egypt, Arab Rep. of	Mean	51.3	−0.42	−3.8	4.2	1.4
	Standard deviation	69.3	0.69	4.6	6.1	2.1
	Minimum	2.6	−4.67	−33.8	0.1	0.0
	Maximum	474.3	−0.01	−0.3	44.1	15.1
Iran, Islamic Rep. of	Mean	38.7	−0.42	−3.8	4.2	1.4
	Standard deviation	52.1	0.70	4.7	6.0	2.1
	Minimum	2.0	−4.73	−34.1	0.1	0.0
	Maximum	358.1	−0.01	−0.3	43.8	15.0
Jordan	Mean	33.6	−0.35	−3.2	3.7	1.3
	Standard deviation	46.8	0.59	3.9	5.3	1.8
	Minimum	1.2	−4.08	−27.6	0.1	0.0
	Maximum	324.5	−0.01	−0.2	38.2	13.2
Lebanon	Mean	30.0	−0.45	−4.4	4.6	1.5
	Standard deviation	38.5	0.72	5.4	6.7	2.2
	Minimum	2.1	−4.87	−39.3	0.1	0.0
	Maximum	265.8	−0.02	−0.4	48.3	15.9
Morocco	Mean	39.5	−0.42	−4.0	4.3	1.4
	Standard deviation	52.0	0.68	4.8	6.1	2.1
	Minimum	2.2	−4.62	−34.3	0.1	0.0
	Maximum	354.5	−0.01	−0.3	43.8	15.0
Tunisia	Mean	54.0	−0.44	−4.2	4.4	1.4
	Standard deviation	70.7	0.71	5.0	6.3	2.1
	Minimum	3.4	−4.78	−36.3	0.1	0.0
	Maximum	479.7	−0.01	−0.3	45.3	14.9
Yemen, Rep. of	Mean	36.5	−0.34	−2.9	3.6	1.3
	Standard deviation	51.3	0.58	3.6	5.3	1.9
	Minimum	1.3	−4.04	−25.7	0.1	0.1
	Maximum	358.5	−0.01	−0.2	38.1	14.1

Note: pvGDP, present value of gross domestic product.
Source: Author's calculations.

FIGURE A.1

Distribution of GDP Losses (2000–25) Resulting from the HIV/AIDS Epidemic

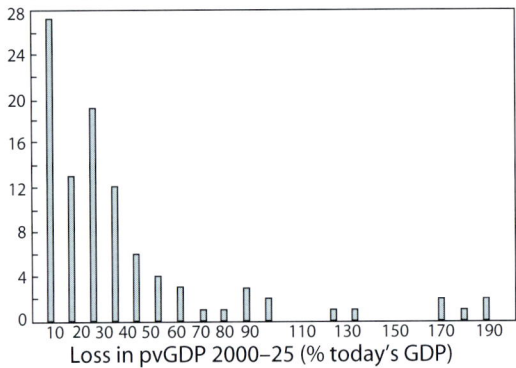

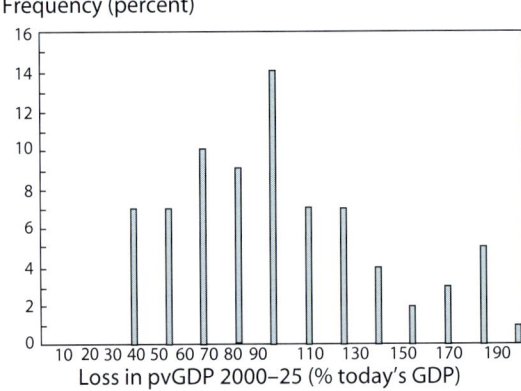

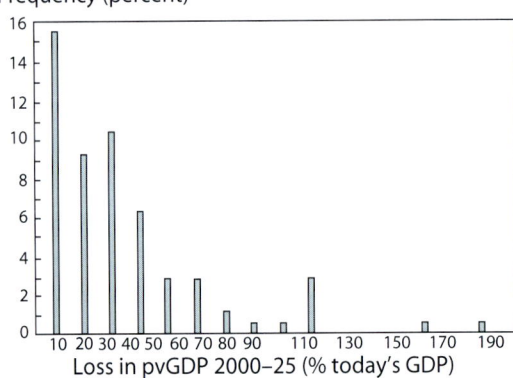

FIGURE A.1 (continued)

Iran, Islamic Rep. of

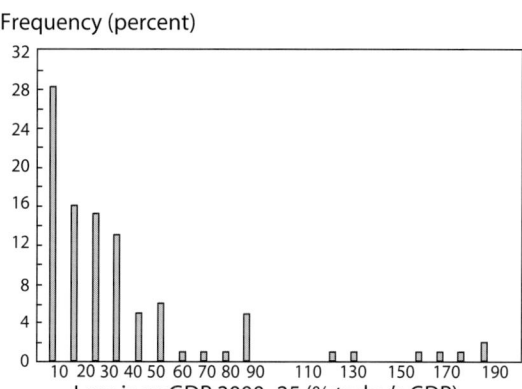

Jordan

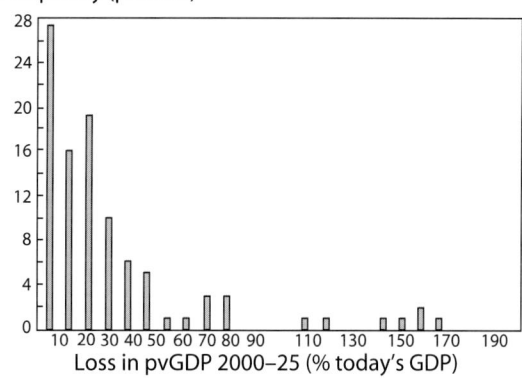

Lebanon

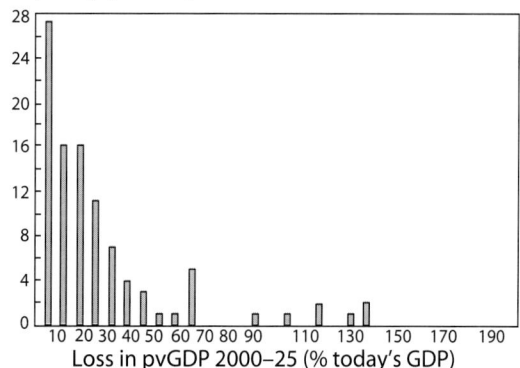

FIGURE A.1 (continued)

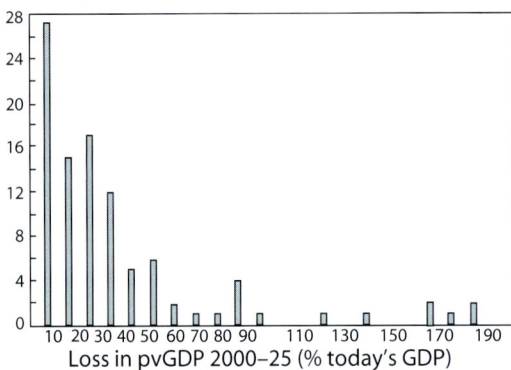

Morocco

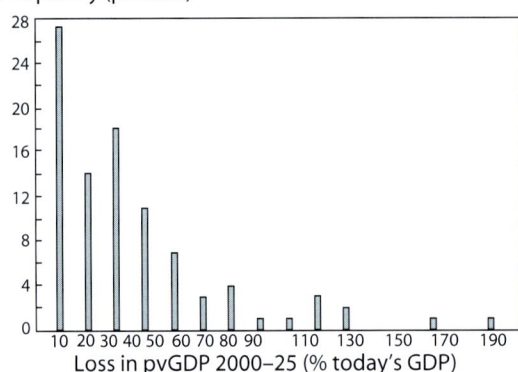

Tunisia

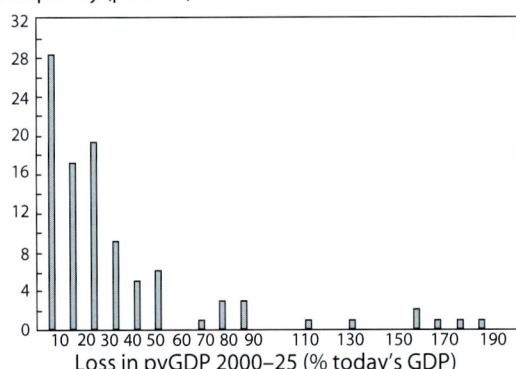

Yemen, Rep. of

FIGURE A.2

Distribution of Reductions in the GDP Growth Rate (2000–25) Resulting from the HIV/AIDS Epidemic

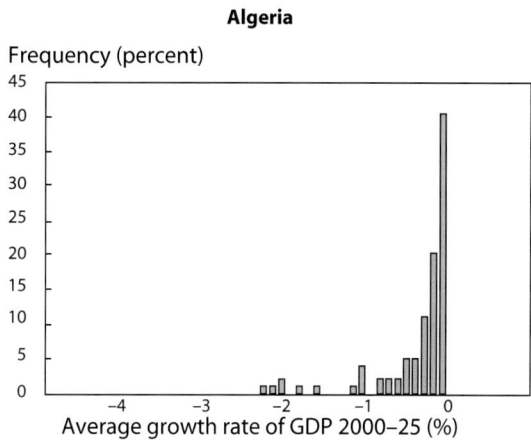

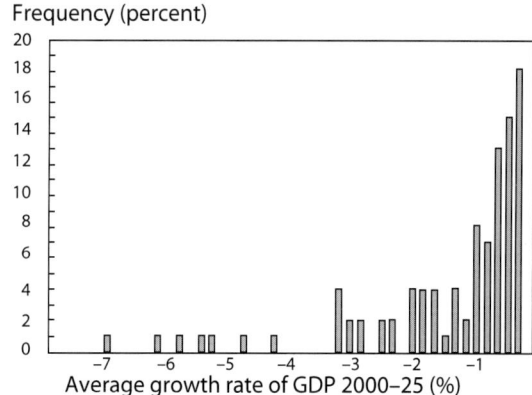

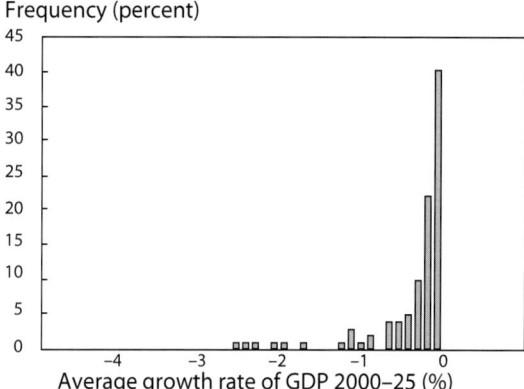

FIGURE A.2 (continued)

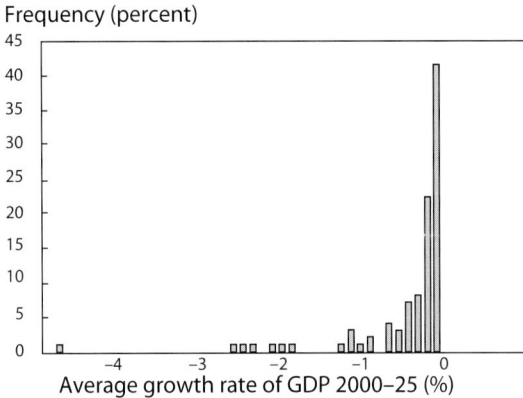

Iran, Islamic Rep. of

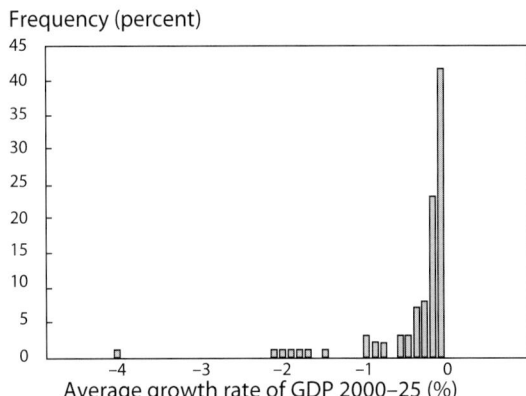

Jordan

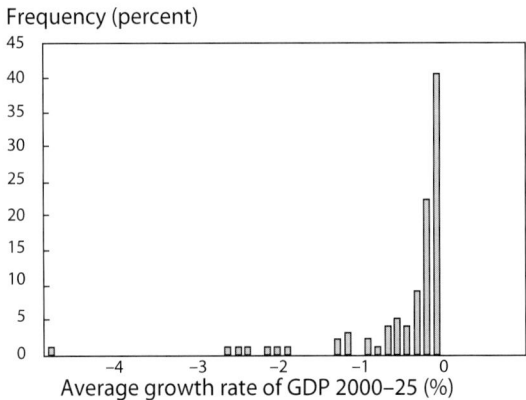

Lebanon

FIGURE A.2 (continued)

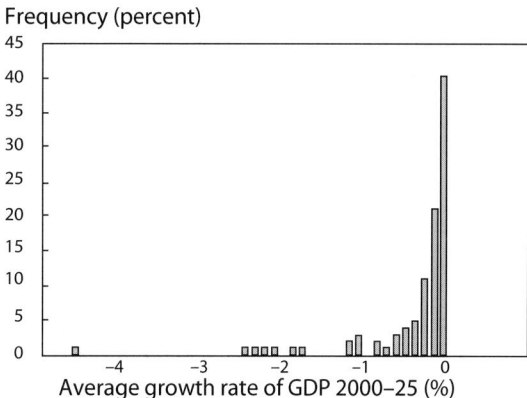

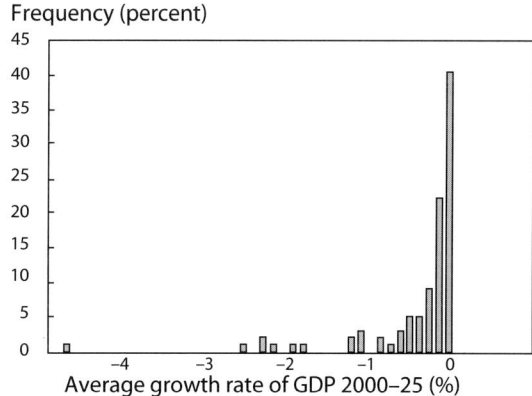

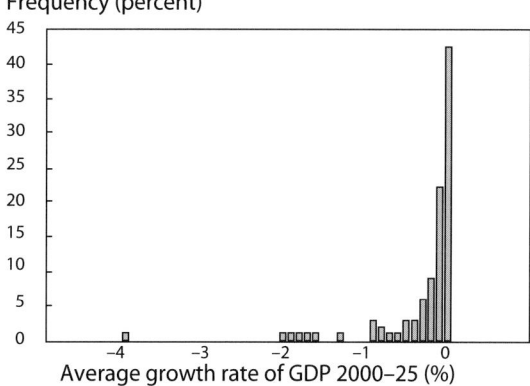

Distribution of Reductions in the Labor Force in 2025

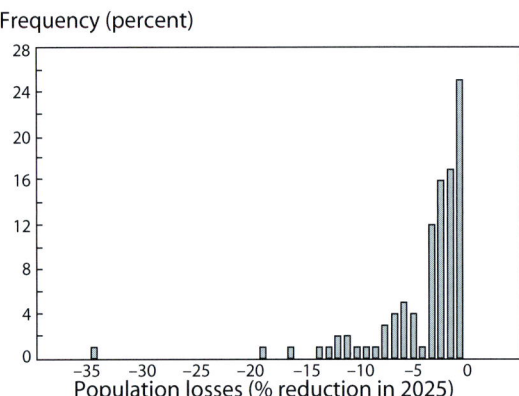

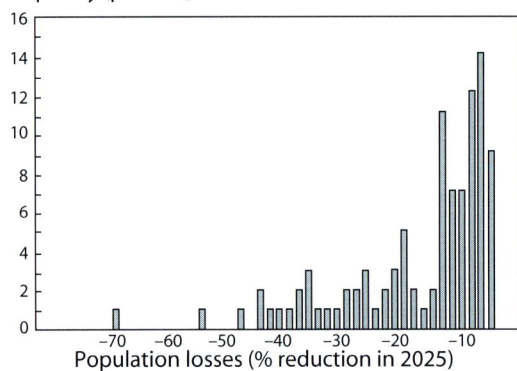

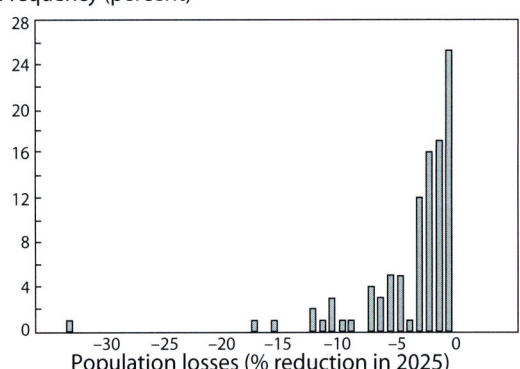

FIGURE A.3 (continued)

Iran, Islamic Rep. of

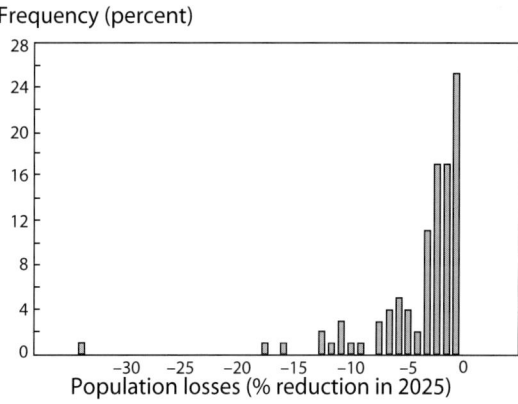

Jordan

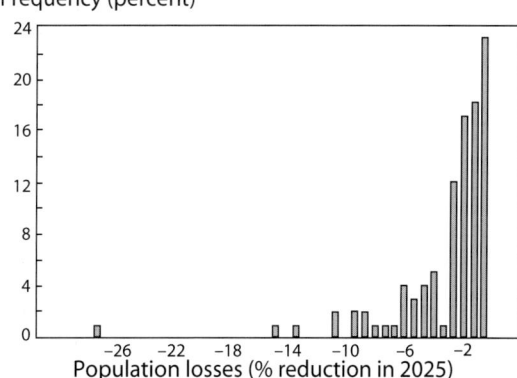

Lebanon

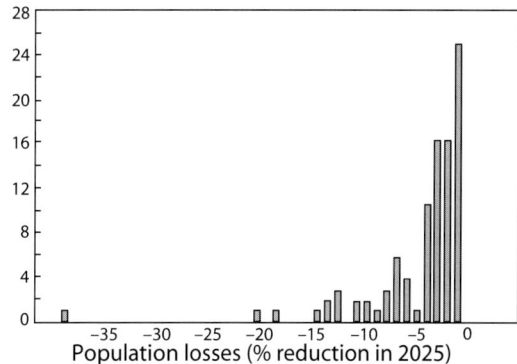

FIGURE A.3 (continued)

Morocco

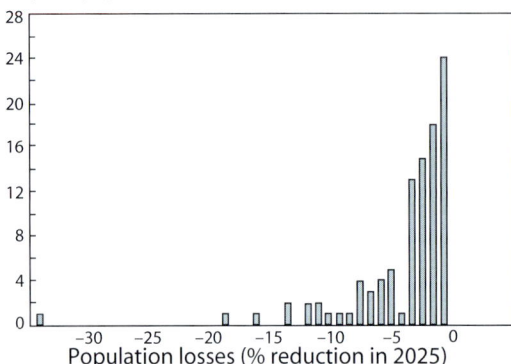

Tunisia

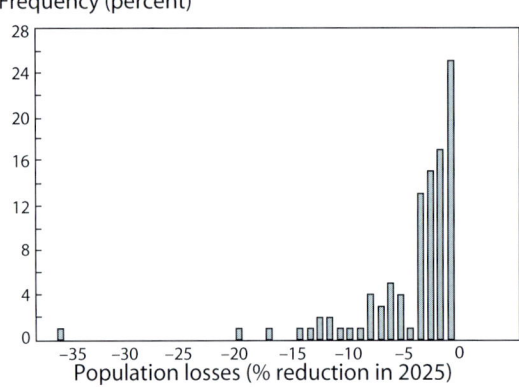

Yemen, Rep. of

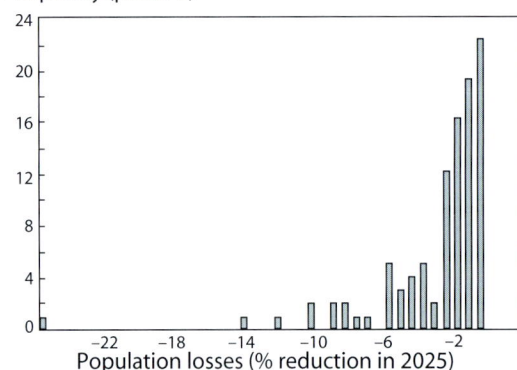

Distribution of the HIV/AIDS Prevalence Level in 2015

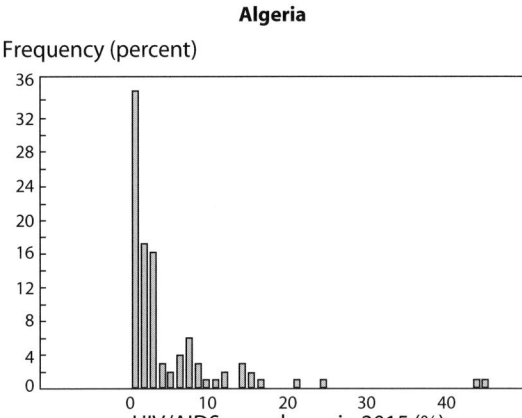

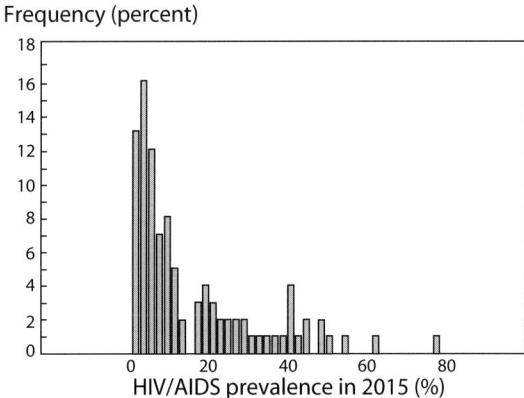

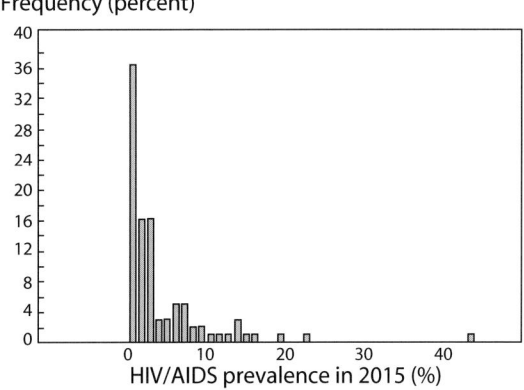

FIGURE A.4 (continued)

Iran, Islamic Rep. of

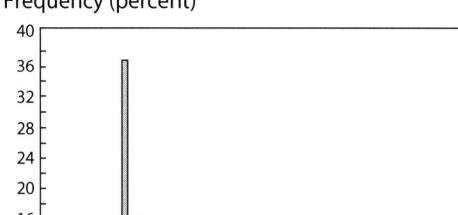

Jordan

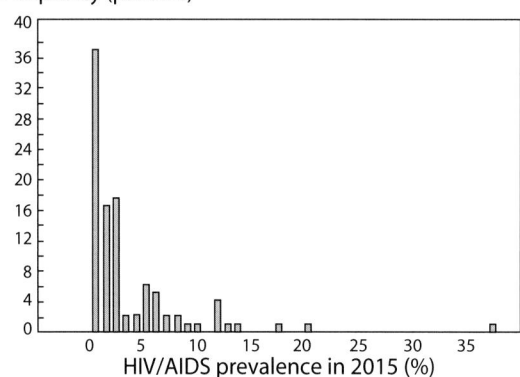

Lebanon

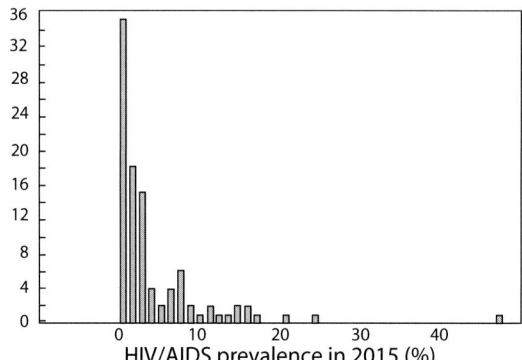

FIGURE A.4 (continued)

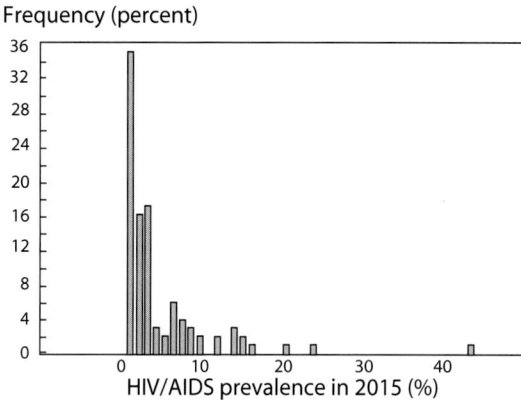

Morocco

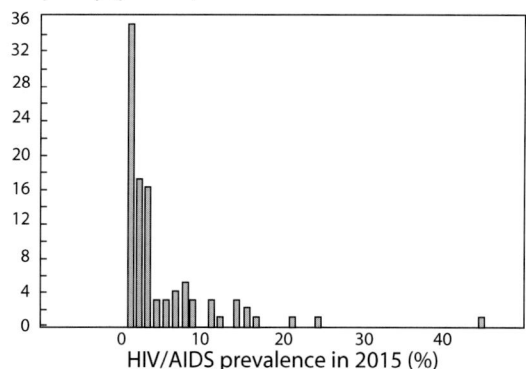

Tunisia

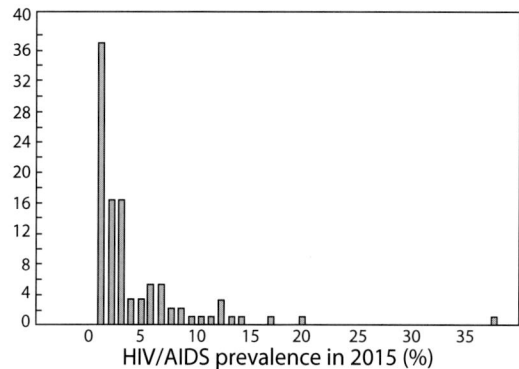

Yemen, Rep. of

Distribution of HIV/AIDS-Related Health Expenditures in 2015

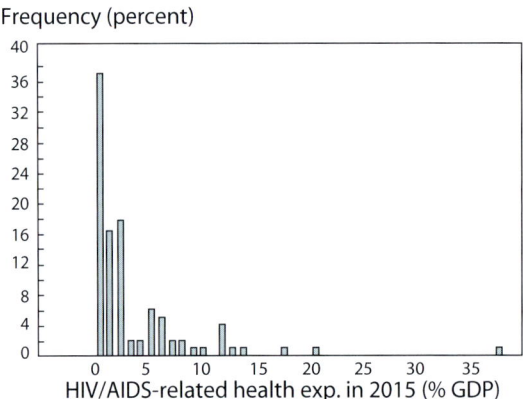

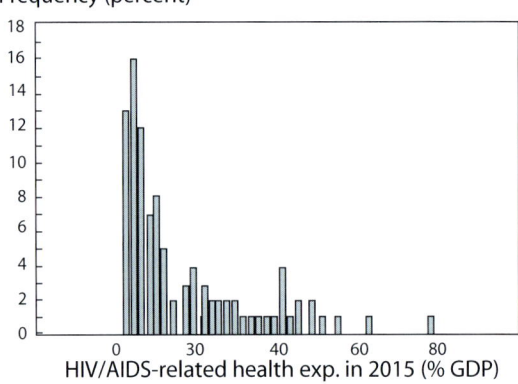

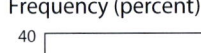

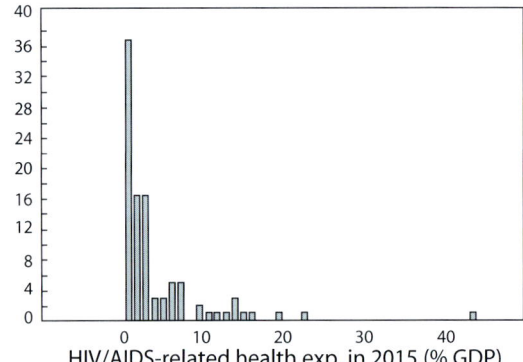

FIGURE A.5 (continued)

Iran, Islamic Rep. of

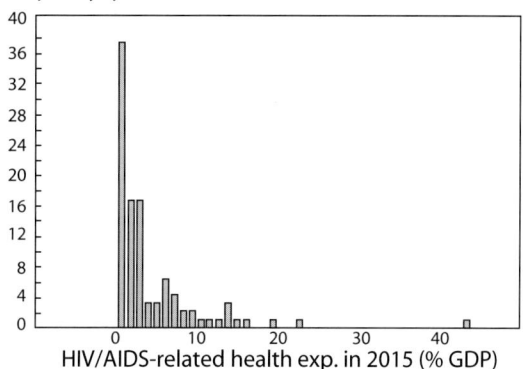

Jordan

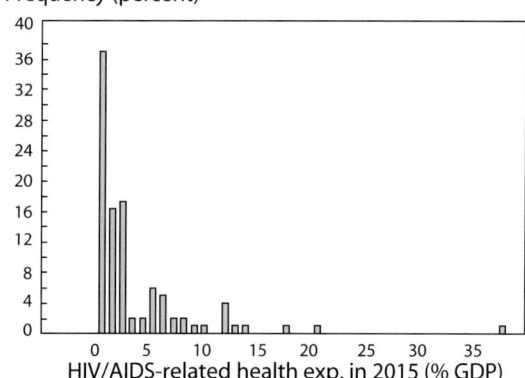

Lebanon

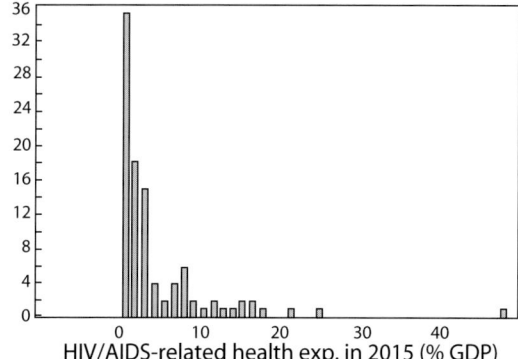

FIGURE A.5 (continued)

Morocco

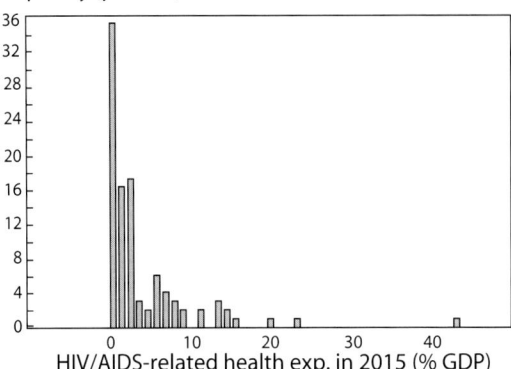

Frequency (percent)

HIV/AIDS-related health exp. in 2015 (% GDP)

Tunisia

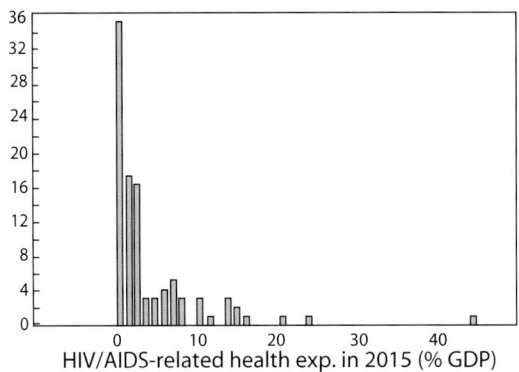

Frequency (percent)

HIV/AIDS-related health exp. in 2015 (% GDP)

Yemen, Rep. of

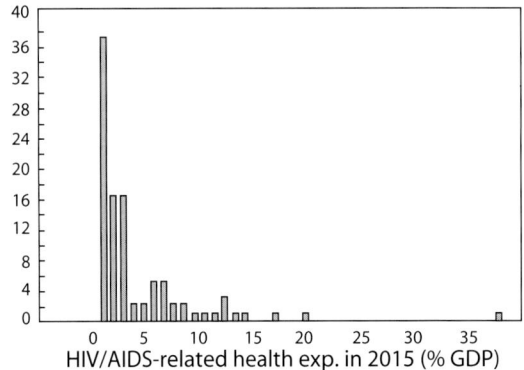

Frequency (percent)

HIV/AIDS-related health exp. in 2015 (% GDP)

Savings Resulting from Increasing Access to Condoms and Clean Needles for IDUs

We focus on two classical interventions: condoms distribution and expanding access to safe needles for IDUs. As discussed in the introduction to this book, heterosexual transmission and transmission through the sharing of infected needles among IDUs are two of the major mechanisms that could sustain the development of the epidemic.

To implement these policies, we affect the parameters dU (equation 12) and dF (equation 14), which are, respectively, the reduction in the probability of sharing a needle and an increase in the probability of using a condom. To evaluate the importance of the timing of the intervention, we also look at two different implementation times. The total costs of these interventions are given by:

$$cost(dF, dU, s) = \sum_{t=s}^{T} \rho \left[sex(t).dF.p_c + drugs(t).dU.p_n \right]$$

where s is the time when the policy is in effect, $sex(.)$ is a function giving the total number of sexual contacts, $drug(.)$ is a function given the total number of needles consumed (both defined on the basis of equations 12 and 14), and p_c and p_n are, respectively, the average costs of distributing a condom and a needle.

The two policies simulated in this exercise are presented in table A.8. In both cases, dU is set equal to 0.20 (that is, the probability of sharing a needle is reduced by 20 percentage points) and dF is set equal to 0.30 (the probability of using a condom increases by 30 percentage points). The first case sets s = 1 (that is, the policy is implemented immediately), while the second case sets s = 5 (the policy is implemented after five years). Since we prefer to underestimate benefits and overestimate costs, we work with high-end estimates from the literature. Thus, we assume that the average cost of distributing a condom is equal to US$0.5 while the average cost of distributing a needle is US$1.5 (see table A.9).

TABLE A.8

Two Classical Interventions: Distributing Condoms and Needles

	Policy A	Policy B
Increase in condom use (dF) (percent)	30	30
Reduction in needle sharing (dU) (percent)	20	20
Year when the policy is implemented (s)	1	5
Average cost of condom in US$ (p_c)	0.5	0.5
Average cost of needle in US$ (p_n)	1.5	1.5

Source: Authors' design.

Unit Costs for Needle Distribution Intervention

Input	Cost	Unit
Cost of needle and syringe	0.1	per unit
Rent for drop-in center	165	month
Electricity for drop-in center	35	month
Supervisor for drop-in center	3,000	year
Cost distributor	2	day

Source: Jenkins, Rahman, and others 2001.

We assume that all costs are directly subtracted from GDP.[7] For each sampled point in the parameter space, we then recompute the same four output variables that are in the nonintervention case. The results are summarized in tables A.10 and A.11.

TABLE A.10

Output Variables under Policy Interventions

Country	Statistic	pvGDP [2000–25] loss (percentage of today's GDP)	Average GDP growth rate, 2000–25 (percent)	Population change, 2025 (percent)	HIV prevalence, 2015 (percent)	Health expenditures, 2015 (percentage of GDP)
Algeria	Mean	19.5	−0.1	−1.4	1.3	0.4
	Standard deviation	21.1	0.2	1.7	2.0	0.7
	Minimum	2.8	−1.8	−12.4	0.0	0.0
	Maximum	171.3	0.0	0.0	15.3	5.1
Djibouti	Mean	93.5	−0.6	−8.4	6.0	2.1
	Standard deviation	59.7	0.6	6.1	7.3	2.6
	Minimum	31.5	−4.5	−39.8	0.2	0.1
	Maximum	422.9	−0.1	−2.9	45.2	16.0
Egypt, Arab Rep. of	Mean	23.2	−0.1	−1.3	1.2	0.4
	Standard deviation	27.2	0.2	1.6	1.9	0.6
	Minimum	2.5	−2.0	−11.7	0.0	0.0
	Maximum	222.0	0.0	0.1	14.4	4.9
Iran, Islamic Rep. of	Mean	17.7	−0.1	−1.3	1.1	0.4
	Standard deviation	20.5	0.2	1.6	1.8	0.6
	Minimum	2.1	−2.0	−11.8	0.0	0.0
	Maximum	167.3	0.0	0.1	14.3	4.8
Jordan	Mean	17.1	−0.1	−1.0	1.0	0.3
	Standard deviation	18.2	0.2	1.3	1.6	0.5
	Minimum	2.4	−1.7	−9.3	0.0	0.0
	Maximum	147.1	0.0	0.0	12.1	4.1
Lebanon	Mean	12.4	−0.1	−1.5	1.2	0.4
	Standard deviation	15.1	0.2	1.8	2.1	0.7
	Minimum	1.3	−2.1	−13.9	0.0	0.0
	Maximum	123.8	0.0	0.1	16.3	5.3
Morocco	Mean	18.5	−0.1	−1.3	1.2	0.4
	Standard deviation	20.6	0.2	1.6	1.8	0.6
	Minimum	2.3	−1.9	−11.8	0.0	0.0
	Maximum	165.4	0.0	0.1	14.2	4.8
Tunisia	Mean	21.0	−0.1	−1.4	1.2	0.4
	Standard deviation	26.9	0.2	1.7	1.9	0.6
	Minimum	1.9	−2.0	−12.6	0.0	0.0
	Maximum	217.8	0.0	0.1	14.8	4.8
Yemen, Rep. of	Mean	37.7	−0.1	−1.0	1.1	0.4
	Standard deviation	25.9	0.2	1.2	1.6	0.6
	Minimum	6.6	−1.8	−8.9	0.0	0.0
	Maximum	208.1	0.0	0.0	12.3	4.5

Note: GDP, gross domestic product; pvGDP, present value of gross domestic product.
Source: Authors' calculations.

TABLE A.11

Output Variables if Policy Intervention Is Postponed for Five Years

Country	Statistic	pvGDP [2000–25] loss (percentage of today's GDP)	Average GDP growth rate, 2000–25 (percent)	Population change, 2025 (percent)	HIV prevalence, 2015 (percent)	Health expenditures, 2015 (percentage of GDP)
Algeria	Mean	28.6	−0.2	−2.4	2.1	0.7
	Standard deviation	30.3	0.3	2.6	3.1	1.1
	Minimum	4.0	−2.5	−19.3	0.0	0.0
	Maximum	236.4	0.0	−0.1	23.3	7.9
Djibouti	Mean	120.6	−0.8	−11.7	8.8	3.1
	Standard deviation	81.8	0.8	8.7	10.2	3.6
	Minimum	33.0	−5.4	−52.4	0.3	0.1
	Maximum	524.7	−0.1	−3.3	57.9	20.6
Egypt, Arab Rep.	Mean	34.5	−0.2	−2.2	2.0	0.7
	Standard deviation	38.7	0.3	2.5	3.0	1.0
	Minimum	4.2	−2.7	−18.4	0.1	0.0
	Maximum	305.6	0.0	−0.1	22.3	7.6
Iran, Islamic Rep. of	Mean	26.3	−0.2	−2.2	2.0	0.7
	Standard deviation	29.3	0.3	2.5	2.9	1.0
	Minimum	3.2	−2.7	−18.5	0.0	0.0
	Maximum	231.0	0.0	−0.1	22.1	7.5
Jordan	Mean	24.3	−0.2	−1.8	1.7	0.6
	Standard deviation	26.0	0.3	2.1	2.5	0.9
	Minimum	2.8	−2.2	−14.6	0.0	0.0
	Maximum	202.3	0.0	0.0	18.6	6.4
Lebanon	Mean	19.5	−0.2	−2.6	2.2	0.7
	Standard deviation	21.9	0.3	2.9	3.3	1.1
	Minimum	2.5	−2.9	−21.8	0.1	0.0
	Maximum	173.3	0.0	−0.1	25.1	8.2
Morocco	Mean	27.5	−0.2	−2.3	2.0	0.7
	Standard deviation	29.5	0.3	2.6	3.0	1.0
	Minimum	3.6	−2.6	−18.6	0.0	0.0
	Maximum	229.1	0.0	0.0	22.1	7.5
Tunisia	Mean	33.2	−0.2	−2.4	2.1	0.7
	Standard deviation	38.9	0.3	2.7	3.1	1.0
	Minimum	4.0	−2.7	−19.7	0.0	0.0
	Maximum	303.7	0.0	−0.1	23.0	7.5
Yemen, Rep. of	Mean	44.9	−0.2	−1.7	1.7	0.6
	Standard deviation	34.6	0.3	1.9	2.5	0.9
	Minimum	6.9	−2.3	−13.8	0.0	0.0
	Maximum	267.2	0.0	−0.1	18.7	6.9

Note: GDP. Gross domestic product.; pvGDP, present value of gross domestic product.
Source: Authors' calculations.

Notes

1. Research has shown that beyond the psychological impacts, among low-income populations, the death of one parent is associated with a deterioration of nutritional status and lower school enrollment rates (Ainsworth and Koda 1993).

2. The implicit assumption is that the consumption of health services to treat AIDS patients is included in the consumption bundle.

3. Notice that as long as t<1, then $\delta U/\delta N = (1 + \tau)N^\tau C^\tau + N^{1+\tau} \tau C^{t-1}$ $\delta C/\delta N > 0$, therefore a reduction in N, as a result of HIV/AIDS, implies a welfare loss.

4. It has been estimated that in the world, three of four new infections are transmitted through sexual intercourse. The exchange of needles among drug users is the second cause of transmission in the world, although in China and Southeast Asia (except Thailand), it is the number one cause. In the case of Argentina and Brazil, needle exchange among drug users explains 25 percent to 35 percent of total new infections.

5. Estimates in the case of Thailand suggest that the probability of transmission from a woman to a man is more on the order of 3 percent to 6 percent. It is also important to note that the probability of transmission is higher during the first weeks of infection and is also influenced by the type of virus. VIH-1 is more easily transmitted than VIH-2.

6. AVERT, despite its simple formulation, has been shown to produce reasonable forecasts of infections averted as a result of interventions, such as increasing condom use or reducing the prevalence of STDs.

7. At the macro level this is not necessarily the case, since the production and distribution of condoms and needles can also contribute to GDP. A more realistic approach, but less conservative, would have been to look at the distortionary effects of reallocating resources to the (production and/or importation) and distribution of needles and condoms.

References

The word *processed* describes informally reproduced works that may not be commonly available through libraries.

Abdelmajid, Ben Hmida. 1999. « Chapitre 1. Situation épidémiologique des maladies sexuellement transmissibles. » Les 7èmes JNSP/DSSB/99. Department of Preventive Medicine, Faculty of Medicine, Tunis. Processed.

Abid, M., C. C. Luo, S. Sekkat, N. De Latore, H. Mansour, D. Holloman-Candal, M. Rayfield, and A. Benslimane. 1998. "Characterization of the V3 Region of HIV Type 1 Isolates from Morocco." *AIDS Res Hum Retroviruses* 14(15):1387–89.

Aghanashinikar, P. N., S. H. al-Dhahry, H. A. al-Marhuby, M. R. Buhl, A. S. Daar, and M. K. Al-Hasani. 1992. "Prevalence of Hepatitis B, Hepatitis Delta, and Human Immunodeficiency Virus Infections in Omani Patients with Renal Diseases." *Transplant Proc* 24(5):1913–14.

Ainsworth, M., and G. Koda. 1993. "The Impact of Adult Deaths from AIDS and Other Causes on School Enrollment in Tanzania." Paper presented at the annual meeting of the Population Association of America, Cincinnati, Ohio, April 1–3, 1993.

Ainsworth, M., and M. Over. 1994. "AIDS and African Development." *World Bank Researcher Observer* 9(2):203–40.

Al-Haddad, M. K., B. Z. Baig, and R. A. Ebrahim. 1997. "Epidemiology of HIV and AIDS in Bahrain." *J Commun Dis* 29(4):321–28.

Al-Haddad, M. K., A. S. Khashaba, B. Z. Baig, and S. Khalfan. 1994. "HIV Antibodies among Intravenous Drug Users in Bahrain." *J Commun Dis* 26(3):127–32.

Ali, K. A. 1996. "Notes on Rethinking Masculinities: An Egyptian Case." In S. Zeidenstein and K. Moore, eds., *Learning about Sexuality*, pp. 98–109. New York: Population Council and Women's Health Coalition.

Al-Jowder, Somaya. 2001. "Bahrain Report." Prepared for the World Health Organization 11th Intercountry Meeting of National AIDS and STD Program Managers, Casablanca, July 2001.

Al-Mahroos, F. T., and A. Ebrahim. 1995. "Prevalence of Hepatitis B, Hepatitis C, and Human Immune Deficiency Virus Markers among Patients with Hereditary Haemolytic Anaemias." *Ann Trop Paediatr* 15(2):121–28.

Al Mulla, K. M. A., R. N. H. Pugh, M. M. Hossain, and R. H. Behrens. 1996. "Travel-Related AIDS Awareness among Young Gulf Arab Men." *J Travel Med* 3(4):224–26.

Al-Nozha, M. M., A. R. al-Frayh, M. al-Nasser, and S. Ramia. 1995. "Horizontal versus Vertical Transmission of Human Immunodeficiency Virus Type 1 (HIV-1): Experience from Southwestern Saudi Arabia." *Trop Geogr Med* 47(6):293–95.

Al-Owaish, R. A., S. Anwar, P. Sharma, and S. F. Shah. 2000. "HIV/AIDS Prevalence among Male Patients in Kuwait." *Saudi Med J* 21(9):852–59.

Al-Owaish, R., M. A. Moussa, S. Anwar, H. al-Shoumer, and P. Sharma. 1999. "Knowledge, Attitudes, Beliefs, and Practices about HIV/AIDS in Kuwait." *AIDS Educ Prev* 11(2):163–73.

Al-Qadhi, Hatem. 2001. "A Silent Threat in Yemen: Confronting HIV/AIDS Choices." United Nations Development Programme.

Al-Qutob, Raeda, Saleh Mawajdeh, Laila Nawar, Slama Saidi, and Firas Raad. 1998. "Assessing the Quality of Reproductive Health Services." Policy Series in Reproductive Health No. 5. Population Council, Cairo.

Al-Sheikh, I. H., A. Rahi, and M. al-Khalifa. 1999. "Mutant Chemokine Receptor (CCR-5) and Its Relevance to HIV Infection in Arabs." *Emerg Infect Dis* 5(1):183–85.

Althaus, Frances. 1997. Special Report. "Female Circumcision: Rite of Passage or Violation of Rights?" *International Family Planning Perspectives* 23(3).

Amini, S., M. F. Mahmoodi, S. Andalibi, and A. A. Solati. 1993. "Sero-epidemiology of Hepatitis B, Delta, and Human Immunodeficiency Virus Infections in Hamadan Province, Iran: A Population-Based Study." *J Trop Med Hyg* 96(5):277–87.

Amnesty International. 2001a. "Egypt 2000, POL 10/001/201." (Web).

———. 2001b. "Middle East and North Africa Regional Update." (Web).

Anderson, J. W. 2001. "Iran's Cultural Backlash, Public Floggings Take Aim at Western Reforms." *Washington Post* Foreign Service, Thursday, August 16, 2001, p. A1.

Anderson, R. 1996. "The Spread of HIV and Sexual Mixing Patterns." In Jonathan Mann and Daniel Tarantola, eds., *AIDS in the World II: Global Dimensions, Social Roots, and Responses. The Global AIDS Policy Coalition.* New York: Oxford University Press.

Aqaie, Faramarz Seyyed. 2001. "The Drug War: All Are in Charge, No One Is Responsible." *Iran Daily* (Tehran), July 26, p. 5, and July 28, p. 5.

Arbesser, C., H. Bashiribod, and W. Sixl. 1987. "Serological Examinations of HIV-I in Iran." *J Hyg Epidemiol Microbiol Immunol* 31 (Suppl 4):504–05.

As'ad, A., and R. Al-Azzeh. 2001. "Jordan Country Report." Prepared for the WHO 11th Intercountry Meeting of National AIDS and STD Program Managers, Casablanca, July 2001.

Attia, M. A. 1998. "Prevalence of Hepatitis B and C in Egypt and Africa." *Antiviral Therapy* 3(Suppl 3):1–9.

Bakir, T. M., K. M. Kurbaan, I. al Fawaz, and S. Ramia. 1995. "Infection with Hepatitis Viruses (B and C) and Human Retroviruses (HTLV-1 and HIV) in Saudi Children Receiving Cycled Cancer Chemotherapy." *J Trop Pediatr* 41(4):206–09.

Ba-Omer, A. A. 2001. "HIV/AIDS/STD Situation and Management in Oman." Presentation prepared for the WHO 11th Intercountry

Meeting of National AIDS and STD Program Managers, Casablanca, July 2001.

———. 2002. "Reported AIDS Cases-Oman." Sultanate of Oman.

BBC. 2001. "Call for Iranian Anti-AIDS Campaign." Sunday, July 29, 2001.

Beegle, Kathleen. 1996." The Impact of Prime-Age Adult Mortality on Labor Supply." Michigan State University, East Lansing. Processed.

Bell, C., S. Devarajan, and H. Gersbach. 2003. "The Economic Impact of Health Shocks on Growth." World Bank. Processed.

Benjelloun, S., B. Bahbouhi, S. Sekkat, A. Bennani, N. Hda, and A. Benslimane. 1996. "Anti-HCV Seroprevalence and Risk Factors of Hepatitis C Virus Infection in Moroccan Population Groups." *Res Virol* 147(4):247–55.

Ben Said, Amel. 2001a. « Point sur la situation épidémiologique de l'infection a VIH/SIDA en Tunisie. » Processed.

———. 2001b. "National AIDS and STDs Program in Tunisia." Presentation prepared for the WHO 11th Intercountry Meeting of National AIDS and STD Program Managers, Casablanca, July 2001.

Ben Yahia, C. 2000. « Programme Jeunes et Santé de la Reproduction. » Office National de la Famille et de la Population. Processed.

Bernvil, S. S., K. Sheth, M. Ellis, H. Harfi, M. Halim, A. Kariem, and V. Andrews. 1991. "HIV Antibody Screening in a Saudi Arabian Blood Donor Population: 5 Years' Experience." *Vox Sang* 61(1):71–73.

Biggs, T., and M. Shah. 1996. "The Impact of the AIDS Epidemic on African Firms." Background Paper. World Bank, Washington, D.C.

Bint Talal, B. 1996. "Arab Women and the Labor Market." *World of Work* (16):24–25.

Blanchet, T. 2002. "Beyond Borders." United States Agency for International Development, Dhaka.

Bloom, D., and A. Mahal. 1995. "Does the AIDS Epidemic Really Threaten Economic Growth?" Working Paper No. 5148. National Bureau of Economic Research, Cambridge, Mass.

Bollinger, L., J. Stover, and D. Nalo. 1999. "The Economic Impact of AIDS in Kenya." The Futures Group International, Glastonbury, Conn. Processed.

Bonnel, René. 2000. "HIV/AIDS: Does It Increase or Decrease Growth?" *South African Journal of Economics.*

Bouakaz, R. 1998. « Ministère de la Santé et de la Population, Direction de la Prévention, Institut National de Santé Publique. » Santé Sud. Processed.

——— 2000. « Migration et SIDA au Sud Algérien: Cas de Tamanrasset. » La Wilaye de Tamanrasset. Processed.

Boudghene-Stambouli, O., A. Merad-Boudia, and A. Aissa-Mamoun. 1992. "The Reappearance of Chancroid in Algeria." *Bull Soc Pathol Exot* 85(4):276–78.

Bourqia, R. 1992. "The Woman's Body: Strategy of Illness and Fertility in Morocco." In Ismail Sirageldin and Robb Davis, eds., *Towards More Efficacy in Women's Health and Child Survival Strategies: Combining Knowledge for Practical Solutions.* Report of the Johns Hopkins University–Ford Foundation Regional Workshop, Cairo, Egypt, December 2–4, 1990; Baltimore, Md., Johns Hopkins University, School of Hygiene and Public Health, Department of Population Dynamics, pp. 131–144.

Boushaba, A., and H. Hammich. 2000. "Outreach-Based Prevention in Morocco among Men Involved in Sex Work. HIV and AIDS in Africa." *Infothek*, pp. 1–3. *UNAIDS Best Practice Digest* (Web).

Boushaba, A., O. Tawil, L. Imane, and H. Himmich. 1999. "Marginalization and Vulnerability: Male Sex Work in Morocco." In Peter Aggleton, ed., *Men Who Sell Sex. International Perspectives on Male Sex work and AIDS*, pp. 263–74. London: UCL Press.

Brunger, W. 1996. "Country Watch: Comoros and Morocco." *AIDS/STD Health Promotion Exchange* 4:8–9.

Cacoub, P., V. V. Ohayon, S. Sekkat, B. Dumont, A. Sbai, F. Lunel, A. Benslimane, P. Godeau, and M. I. Archane. 2000. "Epidemiologic and Virologic Study of Hepatitis C Virus Infection in Morocco." *Gastroenterol Clin Biol* 24(2 bis):169–73.

Carr, J. K., M. O. Salminen, J. Albert, E. Sanders-Buell, D. Gotte, D. L. Birx, and F. E. McCutchan. 1998. "Full Genome Sequences of Human Immunodeficiency Virus Type 1 Subtypes G and A/G Inter-Subtype Recombinants." *Virology* 247(1):22–31.

Center for Health Research, University of Indonesia. 2000. *Results of the 1996–1999 Behavioral Surveillance Surveys in Jakarta, Surabaya, and Manado*. Center for Health Research, University of Indonesia.

Central Intelligence Agency (USA). 2000. "World Fact Book. Egypt." (Web).

Central Statistical Organization (CSO) [Yemen] and Macro International Inc. 1998. *Yemen Demographic and Maternal and Child Health Survey, 1997*. Calverton, Md.

Chelala, Cesar. 1998. "Egypt, Other Middle East Countries See Earliest Stage of AIDS Epidemic." *Al Jadid* 4(23).

Cohen, S., and M. Burger. 2000. "Partnering: A New Approach to Sexual and Reproductive Health." Technical Paper No. 3. United Nations Population Fund, New York.

Colley, D. G. 1996. "Ancient Egypt and Today: Enough Scourges to Go Around." *Emerg Infect Dis* 2(4):362–63.

Constantine, N. T., E. Fox, E. A. Abbatte, and J. N. Woody. 1989. "Diagnostic Usefulness of Five Screening Assays for HIV in an East African City Where Prevalence of Infection is Low." *AIDS* 3(5):313–17.

Constantine, N. T., E. Fox, G. Rodier, and E. A. Abbatte. 1992. "Monitoring for HIV-1, HIV-2, HTLV-I Sero-Progression and Sero-Conversion in a Population at Risk in East Africa." *J Egypt Public Health Assoc* 67(5-6):535–47.

Constantine, N. T., M. F. Sheba, E. Fox, J. N. Woody, and E. A. Abbatte. 1990a. "Serological Evidence for Human Immunodeficiency Virus Type 2 in East Africa." *Int J STD AIDS* 1(1):53–54.

Constantine, N. T., M. F. Sheba, D. M. Watts, Z. Farid, and M. Kamal. 1990b. "HIV Infection in Egypt: A Two and a Half Year Surveillance." *J Trop Med Hyg* 93(2):146–50.

Courbage, Y. 1994. "Fertility Transitions in the Mashreq and in the Maghreb: Education, Emigration, and the Diffusion of Ideas." Paper presented at the Population Council Symposium on Family, Gender, and Population Policy: International Debates and Middle Eastern Realities, Cairo, Egypt, February 7–9, 1994. (Popline).

Couzineau, B., J. Bouloumie, P. Hovette, and R. Laroche. 1991. "Prevalence of Infection by the Human Immunodeficiency Virus (HIV) in a Target Population in the Republic of Djibouti." *Med Trop (Mars)* 51(4):485–86.

Cuddington, J. 1993. "Modeling the Macroeconomic Effects of AIDS, with an Application to Tanzania." *World Bank Economic Review* 7(2):173–89.

Cyrillo, D., L. Paulani, and B. Aguirre. 2001. "Direct Costs of AIDS Treatments in Brazil: A Methodological Comparison." Joint United Nations Programme on HIV/AIDS Home Page. Processed.

Daar, A. S. 1991. "Organ Donation—World Experience; the Middle East." *Transplant Proc* 23(5):2505–07.

Dareini, Ali Akbar. 2001. "Iran Confronts Its Sex Industry." Mashhad, Iran, Associated Press, August 13, 2001.

Davis, H. P. 1992. *Unmarried Women and Changing Conceptions of the Self in Sidi Slimane, Morocco.* Ann Arbor, Mich.: University Microfilms International, 1992. Order No. 9306764.

Davis, Susan S., and D. Davis. 1989. *Adolescence in a Moroccan Town: Making Social Sense.* New Brunswick, N.J.: Rutgers University Press.

Department of Statistics (DOS) [Jordan] and Macro International Inc. 1998. *Jordan Population and Family Health Survey, 1997.* Calverton, Md.

Dollar, D., and A. Kraay. 2001. "Growth Is Good for the Poor." Development Research Group. World Bank.

East West Record. 2001. "Kuwait Wages War on Drugs." June 22, 2001.

Egyptian National AIDS Program. 2001. "HIV/AIDS Surveillance in Egypt." Presentation prepared for the WHO 11th Intercountry Meeting of National AIDS and STD Program Managers, Casablanca, July 2001.

El Deeb, Sarah. 2001. "Egyptian Men Sentenced for Gay Sex." Associated Press, November 14, 2001.

El Din, Hassan. 2001. "Egypt Human Rights Report." In *UNDP Human Development Report*. Oxford University Press. (Web).

El-Gawhary, K. 1995. "Sex Tourism in Cairo." *Middle East Report* (September-October).

———. 1998. "Breaking a Social Taboo: AIDS Hotline in Cairo." *Middle East Report* (Spring). Available at http://www.merip.org/mer/mer206/hotline.htm.

Elharti, E., R. Elaouad, S. Amzazi, H. Himmich, Z. Elhachimi, C. Apetrei, J. C. Gluckman, F. Simon, and A. Benjouad. 1997. "HIV-1 Diversity in Morocco." *AIDS* 11(14):1781–83.

El-Hazmi, M. A., and S. Ramia. 1989. "Frequencies of Hepatitis B, Delta, and Human Immune Deficiency Virus Markers in Multitransfused Saudi Patients with Thalassaemia and Sickle-Cell Disease. *J Trop Med Hyg* 92(1):1–5.

Ellis, Randall, Moneer Alam, and Indrani Gupta. 1997. "Health Insurance in India: Prognosis and Prospectus." Boston University, Boston, Mass. Processed.

El Nakib, Mostafa. 2001. "HIV/AIDS Lebanon Country Report." Prepared for the WHO 11th Intercountry Meeting of National AIDS and STD Program Managers, Casablanca, July 2001.

El-Sayed, N. 2002. Egypt Ministry of Health and Population, National AIDS Control Program. PowerPoint presentation entitled "First Consultation of the Regional Advisory Panel on the Impact of Drug Abuse" (RAPID) at the WHO/EMRO meeting held September 23–26, 2002, Cairo.

El-Sayed, N., A. Darwish, M. El-Geneidy, and M. Mehrez. 1994. "Knowledge, Attitude, and Practice of Homosexuals Regarding HIV in Egypt." National AIDS Program, Ministry of Health and Population, Egypt. Processed.

El-Sayed, N., P. Gomatos, C. Beck-Sagué, U. Dietrich, H. von Briesen, S. Osmanov, J. Esparza, R. Arthur, M. Wahdan, and W. Jarvis. 2000. "Epidemic Transmission of Human Immunodeficiency Virus in Renal Dialysis Centers in Egypt." *J Infect Dis* 181:91–97.

El-Sayed, N. M., P. J. Gomatos, G. R. Rodier, T. F. Wierzba, A. Darwish, S. Khashaba, and R. R. Arthur. 1996. "Seroprevalence Survey of Egyptian Tourism Workers for Hepatitis B Virus, Hepatitis C Virus, Human Immunodeficiency Virus, and *Treponema Pallidum* Infections: Association of Hepatitis C Virus Infections with Specific Regions of Egypt." *Am J Trop Med Hyg* 55(2):179–84.

El-Tawila, Sahar. 2000. "Youth in the Population Agenda: Concepts and Methodologies." West Asia and North Africa Meawards Regional Papers No. 44. Population Council, Cairo.

Eltigani, E. 2000. "Changes in Family-Building Patterns in Egypt and Morocco: A Comparative Analysis." *International Family Planning Perspectives* 26(2):73–78.

El-Zanaty, Fatma, and Ann Way. 2001. *Egypt Demographic and Health Survey 2000*. Calverton, Md.: Ministry of Health and Population [Egypt], National Population Council, and ORC Macro.

EMRO. n.d. "Table of Recorded AIDS Cases for Region, 1987–2002." (personal communication).

Essghairi, Rym. 2000. "IPPF Arab World Region. HIV/AIDS in the Arab World." Presentation made at the IPPF HIV/AIDS Working Group Meeting, London, December 2000. Processed.

Etchepare, M. 2001. Programme National de Lutte contre le SIDA et les MST Draft report. World Bank Mission for Health Project Strategy Development, Djibouti.

———. 2002. « Enquête nationale séroprévalence VIH en République de Djibouti. » Processed.

Fam, M. 2001. "Egypt Party Raids Put Focus on Gays." Associated Press, July 16, 2001.

Family Health International. 1998–2000. "Evaluation of Selected Reproductive Health Infections in Various Egyptian Population Groups in Greater Cairo." FHI/MOHP/USAID.

———. 2001a. "What Drives HIV in Asia? A Summary of Trends in Sexual and Drug-Taking Behaviors." FHI/DFID/IMPACT.

———. 2001b. "Effective Prevention Strategies in Low HIV Prevalence Settings. UNAIDS Best Practice Key Materials." FHI/IMPACT/USAID.

———. 2001c. "HIV/AIDS/STI Prevention Program Support Strategy for Jordan." Processed.

Farghaly, A. G., and M. M. Kamal. 1991. "Study of the Opinion and Level of Knowledge about the AIDS Problem among Secondary School Students and Teachers in Alexandria." *J Egypt Public Health Assoc* 66(1–2):209–25.

Faris, R., and A. Shouman. 1994. "Study of the Knowledge, Attitude of Egyptian Health Care Workers towards Occupational HIV Infection." *J Egypt Public Health Assoc* 69(1–2):115–28.

Farza, A. M. 2001. « Rapport de fin de mission d'assistance technique pour la formulation du Plan Stratégique National de Lutte contre le SIDA, 2002–2004 au Maroc, Rabat, Mars-Juin. » Processed.

Feki, S., Z. Rekaya, T. Ben Chaaben, A. Zribi, K. Boukef, and F. Jenhani. 1998. "Determination of T-Lymphocyte Subsets in a North African Population (Tunisia): Establishment of Normal Ranges and Results in HIV-Infected Individuals." *Dis Markers* 14(3):161–64.

Fix, A., M. Abdel-Hamid, R. Purcell, M. Shehata, F. Abdel-Aziz, N. Mikhail, H. El Sebai, M. Nafeh, M. Habib, R. Arthur, S. Emerson, and G. Strickland. 2000. "Prevalence of Antibodies to Hepatitis E in Two Rural Egyptian Communities." *Am J Trop Med Hyg* 62(4):519–23.

Floyd, K., and C. Gilks. 2001. "Cost and Financing Aspects of Providing Anti-Retroviral Therapy: A Background Paper." Joint United Nations Programme on HIV/AIDS Home Page. Processed.

Fox, E., E. A. Abbatte, Said-Salah, N. T. Constantine, G. Rodier, and J. N. Woody. 1989a. "Incidence of HIV Infection in Djibouti in 1988." *AIDS* 3(4):244–45.

Fox, E., E. A. Abbatte, H. H. Wassef, J. N. Woody, Said-Salah, W. Sidrak, and N. T. Constantine. 1989b. "Low Prevalence of HIV Infection in Djibouti—Has the AIDS Epidemic Come to a Stop at the Horn of Africa?" *Trans R Soc Trop Med Hyg* 83(1):103–06.

Fox, E., N. T. Constantine, E. A. Abbatte, Said-Salah, and G. Rodier. 1988. "Low Prevalence of Infection by HTLV-I in Populations at Risk for HIV in Djibouti." *Ann Institut Pasteur Virol* 139(4):443–47.

Fox, E., N. T. Constantine, G. Rodier, and E. A. Abbatte. 1992. "Diagnostic Challenges: Lymphotropic Sero-'Questionables'." *East Afr Med J* 69(10):563–66.

Fox, E., R. L. Haberberger, Jr., E. A. Abbatte, Said-Salah, D. Polycarpe, and N. T. Constantine. 1989. "Observations on Sexually Transmitted Diseases in Promiscuous Males in Djibouti." *J Egypt Public Health Assoc* 64(5–6):561–69.

Garg, S., P. Bhalla, N. Sharma, R. Sahay, A. Puri, R. Saha, P. Sodhani, N. S. Murthy, and M. Mehra. 2001. "Comparisons of Self-Reported Symptoms of Gynecological Morbidity with Clinical and Laboratory Diagnosis in a New Delhi Slum." *Asia-Pacific Pop J* (June):75–92.

GFATM (Global Fund to Fight AIDS, TB and Malaria). 2002. "Yemen Proposal."

Ghannam. Farha. 1997. "Fertile, Plump, and Strong: The Social Construction of the Female Body in Low-Income Cairo." Monographs in Reproductive Health No. 3. Population Council, Cairo.

Ghurayyib, R. 1992. "The Women of the Maghreb." *Al-Raida* 10(57):13–16.

Goodwin, J. 1995. *Price of Honor*. London: Warner Books.

Government of Yemen/United Nations Children's Fund/World Bank/Radda Barnen. 1998. *Children and Women in Yemen: A Situation Analysis* (4 volumes). Sana'a, Republic of Yemen.

Govindasamy, P., and A. Malhotra. 1994. "Aspects of Female Autonomy in Egypt: What Can We Learn from DHS Data?" Presented at the Annual Meeting of the Population Association of America, Miami, Fla., May 5–7, 1994. (Popline).

Groterath, A., and R. Bless. 2002. "Drug Abuse and HIV/AIDS in the Middle East and North Africa. A Situation Assessment." Office on Drugs and Crime, Regional Office for the Middle East and North Africa. Processed.

Gueddána, Nébiha, M. Attia, H. Ben Romdhane, and M. Halayem. 1996. « Les Jeunes au quotidien. » République Tunisienne, Ministère de la Santé Publique, Tunis.

Guenena, Nemat, and Nadia Wassef. 1999. "Unfulfilled Promises: Women's Rights in Egypt." Population Council, Cairo.

Gulf News. 2000. "Health Agency Raises Estimate of AIDS Victims in UAE." Dubai, *Gulf News* Online Edition, January 12, 2000. Available at www.gulfnews.com.

Guman, M., T. al Karmi, M. L. Lukic, and K. Behbehani. 1990. "Detection of HIV-2 Infection in the Gulf Region." *AIDS Res Hum Retroviruses* 6(12):1469–70.

Haacker, Markus. 2001. "The Impact of HIV/AIDS on Economic Growth and Per-Capita Income: A Conceptual Framework." Research Department, International Monetary Fund. Processed.

Hachicha, J., A. Hammami, H. Masmoudi, M. Ben Hmida, H. Karray, M. Kharrat, F. Kammoun, and A. Jarraya. 1995. "Viral Hepatitis C in Chronic Hemodialyzed Patients in Southern Tunisia: Prevalence and Risk Factors. *Ann Med Interne* (Paris) 146(5):295–98.

Haeri, Shahla. n.d. *Law of Desire: Temporary Marriage in Shi'i Iran*. Syracuse, N.Y.: Syracuse University Press. (Popline).

———. 2000. "Temporary Marriage and the State in Iran: An Islamic Discourse on Female Sexuality." In Pinar Ilkkaracen, ed., *Women and Sexuality in Muslim Societies*, pp. 343–62. Istanbul: Women for Women's Human Rights/Kaddinin Insan Haklari Projesi.

Hal, A. A. 1997. "Current Status of Women's Health in the United Arab Emirates." *WIPHN News* (Winter) 22:3.

Hancock, J., D. Nalo, M. Aoko, R. Mutemi, H. Clark, and S. Forsythe. 1996. "The Macroeconomic Impact of AIDS in Kenya." In S. Forsythe and Rau, eds., *AIDS in Kenya*. Arlington: Family Health International, 1996.

Hankins, C., S. Friedman, T. Zafar, and S. Strathdee. 2002. "Transmission and Prevention of HIV and Sexually Transmitted Infections in War Settings: Implications for Current and Future Armed Conflicts." *AIDS* 16:2245–52.

Hassan, N. F., N. M. el Ghorab, M. S. Abdel Rehim, M. S. el Sharkawy, N. M. Sayed, K. Emara, Y. Soltant, M. Sanad, R. G. Hibbs, and R. R. Arthur. 1994. "HIV Infection in Renal Dialysis Patients in Egypt." *AIDS* 8(6):853.

Hawkes, S., L. Morison, S. Foster, K. Gausia, J. Chakraborty, R. W. Peeling, and D. Mabey. 1999. "Reproductive Tract Infections in Women in Low-Income, Low-Prevalence Situations: Assessment of Syndromic Management in Matlab, Bangladesh." *Lancet* 354:1776–81.

Heikel, J., S. Sekkat, F. Bouqdir, H. Rich, B. Takourt, F. Radouani, N. Hda, S. Ibrahimy, and A. Benslimane. 1999. "The Prevalence of Sexually Transmitted Pathogens in Patients Presenting to a Casablanca STD Clinic." *Eur J Epidemiol* 15(8):711–15.

Heise, L., K. Moore, and N. Toubia. 1996. "Defining 'Coercion' and 'Consent' Cross-Culturally." *Siecus Report* 24(2):12–14. Iran.

Helmy, Magdy. 1999. "Female Genital Mutilation in Egypt. Lessons Learned." Cairo: United Nations Children's Fund. Processed.

Hermez, J. 2002. "Experiences in Research, Outreach and the Role of NGOs. Lebanese National AIDS Control Programme." PowerPoint presentation at the WHO/EMRO meeting, First Consultation of the Regional Advisory Panel on the Impact of Drug Abuse (RAPID), Cairo, September 23–26, 2002.

Hmida, S., N. Mojaat, E. Chaouchi, T. Mahjoub, B. Khlass, S. Abid, and K. Boukef. 1995. "HCV Antibodies in Hemodialyzed Patients in Tunisia." *Pathol Biol* (Paris) 43(7):581–83.

Hossini, C. H., D. Tripodi, A. E. Rahhali, M. Bichara, D. Betito, J. P. Curtes, and C. Verger. 2000. "Knowledge and Attitudes of Health Care Professionals with Respect to AIDS and the Risk of Occupational Transmission of HIV in Two Moroccan Hospitals. *Santé* 10(5):315–21.

Huntington, Dale, Laila Nawar, Nahla Abdel-Tawab, Ezzeldin Osman Hassan, and Hala Youssef. 1998. "The Postabortion Caseload in Egyptian Hospitals: A Descriptive Study." *International Family Planning Perspectives* (March).

Ilkkaracen, Pinar, ed. 2000. *Women and Sexuality in Muslim Societies*. Istanbul: Women for Women's Human Rights/Kaddinin Insan Haklari Projesi.

Ingold, François-Rodolphe, and the Lebanese Research Cooperative. 1994. "Rapid Assessment of Illicit Drug Use in Great Beyrouth." United Nations Drug Control Programme, Vienna.

International Center for Research on Women; Development Alternatives; Women, Law, and Development International; AED; Development Associated Inc. 1998. "Women and Development in Jordan: A Review of Current Activities and Future Opportunities." WIDTECH, Washington, D.C.

———. 1999. "Elaborating a Gender Strategy for USAID/Morocco." WIDTECH, Washington, D.C.

International Cooperation for Development/Charitable. 2001. "Society for Social Welfare: Project Proposal: Refugee Health Project-HIV/AIDS." Yemen.

IPPF (International Planned Parenthood Foundation). 2001a. "Empowering Women to Combat HIV: An IPPF Arab World Initiative (Algeria, Djibouti, Mauritania, Sudan, Tunisia)." Grant application to the European Union in response to RFP No. SCRE/110768/C/G. Processed.

———. 2001b. "Meeting the Reproductive Health Needs of Young Adults in the Arab World (Algeria, Jordan, Lebanon, Morocco, Tunisia)." Grant application to the European Union in response to RFP No. SCRE/110768/C/G. Processed.

Iran Daily (Tehran). 2001a. "160 Drug Dealers Arrested in Tehran Park." August 4, 2001.

———. 2001b. "Deadly Disease." Farsi Press Watch, August 4, 2001.

IRNA Zahedan (news agency). 2001. "Fourteen Die in Southeastern Iran from HIV Infection-academic." Sistan va Baluchestan Province, BBC, July 22, 2001.

Islamic Republic of Iran. 2001. "AIDS in the Islamic Republic of Iran." Prepared for the WHO 11th Intercountry Meeting of National AIDS and STD Program Managers, Casablanca, July 2001.

Jemni, L., S. Bahri, M. Saadi, A. Letaif, M. Dhidah, H. Lahdhiri, and S. Bouchoucha. 1991. "AIDS and Tuberculosis in Central Tunisia." *Tunis Med* 69(5):349–52.

Jenkins, C., Shale Ahmed, Habibur Rahman, and M. M. Faisal. 2001. "Male Prostitutes in Dhaka: Risk Reduction through Effective Intervention." Paper presented at the International Conference on AIDS in the Asia-Pacific, Melbourne, October 2001.

Jenkins, C., H. Rahman, T. Saidel, S. Jana, and A. M. Z. Hussain. 2001. "Measuring the Impact of Needle Exchange Programs among Injecting Drug Users though the National Behavioral Surveillance in Bangladesh." *AIDS Education and Prevention* 13(5):452–61.

Kahn, J. 1996. "The Cost-Effectiveness of HIV-Prevention Targeting: How Much More Bang for the Buck?" *Am J Public Health* 86(12):1709–12.

Kalaajieh, W. K. 2000. "Epidemiology of Human Immunodeficiency Virus and Acquired Immunodeficiency Syndrome in Lebanon from 1984 through 1998." *Int J Infect Dis* 4(4):209–13.

Kambou, G., S. Devarajan, and M. Over. 1992. "The Economic Impact of AIDS in an African Country: Simulations with a General Equilibrium Model of Cameroon." *Journal of African Economies* 1(1):109–30.

Kaplan, E., and H. Pollack. 1998. "Allocating HIV Prevention Resources." *Socio-Economic Planning and Science* 21(4):257–63.

Karki, B. B. 2000. "Rapid Assessment among Drug Users in Nepal." *AIDS Watch*, WHO Southeast Asia Region Newsletter on STI, HIV, and TB, May–August 2000. Also in *UNAIDS Best Practice Digest*.

Kassem, S., A. A. el-Nawawy, M. N. Massoud, S. Y. el-Nazar, and E. M. Sobhi. 2000. "Prevalence of Hepatitis C Virus (HCV) Infection and Its Vertical Transmission in Egyptian Pregnant Women and Their Newborns." *J Trop Pediatr* 46(4):231–33.

Kennedy, M., D. O'Reilly, and M. W. Mah. 1998. "The Use of a Quality-Improvement Approach to Reduce Needlestick Injuries in a Saudi Arabian Hospital." *Clin Perform Qual Health Care* 6(2):79–83.

Khaled, L. 1995. "Migration and Women's Status: The Jordan Case." *International Migration* 33(2):235–50.

Khan, S. 1995. "The Silent Killer: AIDS and the Muslim World." *Naz Ki Pukaar* 8 (January).

———. 1996. "Developing Appropriate Strategies." Consultation Meeting of Representatives from Non-Governmental Organizations Working on HIV/AIDS Prevention and Care Issues within Muslim Communities, October 26–29, 1995, Karachi, Pakistan. Final Report, Naz Foundation, submitted to Ford Foundation, New York. Processed.

Khattab, Hind. 1992. "The Silent Endurance: Social Conditions of Women's Reproductive Health in Rural Egypt." United Nations Children's Fund/Population Council, Cairo.

———. 1996. "Women's Perceptions of Sexuality in Rural Gaza." Monographs in Reproductive Health No. 1. Population Council, Cairo.

Khattab, H., H. Zurayk, N. Younis, and O. Kamal. 1996. "Involving Women in a Reproductive Morbidity Study in Egypt." In S. Zeidenstein and K. Moore, eds., *Learning about Sexuality*. New York: Population Council and Women's Health Coalition.

Khattab, Hind, Nabil Younis, and Huda Zurayk. 1999. *Women, Reproduction, and Health in Rural Egypt. The Giza Study.* Cairo: American University of Cairo Press.

Kremer, M. 1996a. "AIDS: The Economic Rationale for Public Intervention." World Bank. Processed.

———. 1996b. "Optimal Subsidies for AIDS Prevention." World Bank. Processed.

Kulwicki, A., and P. S. Cass. 1994. "An Assessment of Arab American Knowledge, Attitudes, and Beliefs about AIDS." *Image J Nurs Sch* 26(1):13–17.

Kuwait National AIDS Program. 2001. "Progress Report of National AIDS Program, State of Kuwait, 2001." Prepared for WHO 11th Intercountry Meeting of National AIDS and STD Program Managers, Casablanca, July 2001.

Lane, S. D. 1992. "Gender and Health in Rural Egyptian Households." In I. Sirageldin and R. Davis, eds., *Towards More Efficacy in Women's Health and Child Survival Strategies: Combining Knowledge for Practical Solutions*. Report of the Johns Hopkins University–Ford Foundation Regional Workshop, Cairo, Egypt, December 2–4, 1990; Baltimore, Md., Johns Hopkins University, School of Hygiene and Public Health, Department of Population Dynamics, August 1992:145–67. (Popline).

Lasky, M., J. L. Perret, M. Peeters, F. Bibollet-Ruche, F. Liegeois, D. Patrel, S. Molinier, C. Gras, and E. Delaporte. 1997. "Presence of Multiple Non-B Subtypes and Divergent Subtype B Strains of HIV-1 in Individuals Infected after Overseas Deployment." *AIDS* 11(1):43–51.

Law, M. 2001. "An HIV Transmission Model." National Center in HIV Epidemiology and Clinical Research, Australia. Processed.

Leighton, C. 1993. "Economic Impacts of the HIV/AIDS Epidemic in African and Asian Settings: Case Studies of Kenya and Thailand." Abt Associates, Bethesda, Md.

———. 1996. "The Direct and Indirect Costs of HIV/AIDS." In Forsythe and Rau, eds., *AIDS in Kenya*. Arlington, Family Health International.

Leonard, G., A. Sangare, M. Verdier, E. Sassou-Guesseau, G. Petit, J. Milan, S. M'Boup, J. L. Rey, J. L. Dumas, J. Hugon, and others.

1990. "Prevalence of HIV Infection among Patients with Leprosy in African Countries and Yemen." *J Acquir Immune Defic Syndr* 3(11):1109–13.

Lewis, A. 2000. "The Macro Implications of HIV/AIDS in South Africa: A Preliminary Assessment." Processed.

Littman, R. J., and D. M. Morens. 1996. "AIDS and AAA in Egypt?" *Emerg Infect Dis* 2(4):363.

MacFarlan, Maitland, and Silvia Sgherri. 2001. "The Macroeconomic Impact of HIV/AIDS in Botswana." International Monetary Fund Working Paper WP/01/80.

Manhart, L. E., A. Dialmy, C. A. Ryan, and J. Mahjour. 2000. "Sexually Transmitted Diseases in Morocco: Gender Influences on Prevention and Health Care Seeking Behavior." *Soc Sci Med* 50(10):1369–83.

Martin, S., B. Kilgallen, A. O. Tsui, K. Maitra, K. K. Singh, and L. Kupper. 1999. "Sexual Behaviors and Reproductive Health Outcomes: Associations with Wife Abuse in India. *JAMA* 282(20).

Massenet, D., and A. Bouh. 1997. "Aspects of Blood Transfusion in Djibouti." *Med Trop (Mars)*57(2):202–05.

Masterson, J., and J. Swanson. 2000. *Female Genital Cutting: Breaking the Silence, Enabling Change*. Washington, D.C.: International Center for Research on Women and the Center for Development and Population Activities.

Mboudjeka, I., B. Bikandou, L. Zekeng, J. Takehisa, Y. Harada, Y. Yamaguchi-Kabata, Y. Taniguchi, E. Ido, L. Kaptue, P. M'pelle, H. J. Parra, M. Ikeda, M. Hayami, and T. Miura. 1999. "Genetic Diversity of HIV-1 Group M from Cameroon and Republic of Congo." *Arch Virol* 144(12):2291–311.

Mehra, Rekha, and Hilary Feldstein. 1998. "Women and Development in Jordan." In *A Review of Current Activities and Future Opportunities*. International Center for Research on Women, WIDTECH, and United States Agency for International Development.

Mernissi, F. 1985. *Beyond the Veil*. London: Al Saqi Books.

———. 2000. "Virginity and Patriarchy." In Pinar Ilkkaracen, ed., *Women and Sexuality in Muslim Societies*, pp. 203–14. Istanbul: Women for Women's Human Rights/Kaddinin Insan Haklari Projesi.

Milder, J. E., and V. M. Novelli. 1992. "Clinical, Social, and Ethical Aspects of HIV-1 Infections in an Arab Gulf State." *J Trop Med Hyg* 95(2):128–31.

Ministère de la Santé/PNLS, de la Jeunesse, de la Promotion de la Femme, de l'Education, ADEPF, and UNICEF. 2001. « Etude des connaissances—attitudes-pratiques des jeunes et leurs participations à la promotion de leurs activités et à la prévention des VIH/SIDA/MST à Djiboutiville. » Processed.

Ministry of Health in collaboration with UNAIDS and WHO. 1999. "Knowledge, Attitudes, Beliefs, and Practices on AIDS in Jordan." The Hashemite Kingdom of Jordan.

Ministry of Health, Djibouti. 2001. "HIV/AIDS Epidemic and Sexually Transmitted Diseases in Djibouti Republic."

Ministry of Health, Sultanate of Oman. 2000. "HIV/AIDS and STI Prevention through Peer Education among Young People in the Sultanate of Oman." HIV/AIDS/STI Prevention and Control Programme.

Ministry of Health, Syrian Arab Republic. 2000. "Development of Community-Based HIV/AIDS Education and Communication for Youths Residing in Slum Areas of Damascus, Syria." National AIDS Program.

Ministry of Health and Population, National AIDS Control Program, Egypt. 2001. "HIV/AIDS Prevention and Control." Processed.

Ministry of Public Health, Tunisia. 2000. "Summary Report for International Forum on the Implementation of the ICPD Program of Action, 1994–1999." National Family and Population Board, Tunis.

———. 2001. « Atelier national de concertation sur la lutte contre le VIH/SIDA en Tunisie. » Processed.

Mohamed, A. E., M. A. al Karawi, and G. A. Mesa. 1997. "Dual Infection with Hepatitis C and B Viruses: Clinical and Histological Study in Saudi Patients." *Hepatogastroenterology* 44(17):1404–06.

Montavon, C., C. Toure-Kane, F. Liegeois, E. Mpoudi, A. Bourgeois, L. Vergne, J. L. Perret, A. Boumah, E. Saman, S. Mboup, E. Delaporte, and M. Peeters. 2000. "Most env and gag Subtype A HIV-1 Viruses Circulating in West and West Central Africa Are Similar to the Prototype AG Recombinant Virus IBNG." *J Acquir Immune Defic Syndr* 23(5):363–74.

Moore, M. 2001. "Once Hidden, Drug Addiction Is Changing Iran. Problem's Impact Challenges Attitudes of a Strict Society." *Washington Post* Foreign Service, July 18, 2001, p. A26.

Morgan-Capner, P., G. A. Holbrook, and J. A. O'Donoghue. 1993. "HIV and Insurance." *BMJ* 307(6907):805.

Morocco National AIDS Program. 2001. "Country Report." Prepared for the WHO 11th Intercountry Meeting of National AIDS and STD Program Managers, Casablanca, July 2001.

Mosbah, F., and C. Ben Yahi. 1998. « Prévention de la toxicomanie et santé sexuelle et reproductive. » Enquête Qualitative sur les Jeunes, Association Tunisienne du Planning Familial.

Muir, Jim. 2002. "Tackling AIDS in Iran." BBC News, March 20, 2002.

Murray, C., and A. Lopez. 1996. "The Global Burden of Disease." In *Global Burden of Disease and Injury Series, Volume 1.* WHO, Harvard School of Public Health, World Bank. Cambridge, Mass.: Harvard University Press.

Murray, S., and W. Roscoe. 1997. *Islamic Homosexualities.* New York: University Press.

Nafeh, M., A. Medhat, M. Shehata, N. Mikhail, Y. Swifee, M. Abdel-Hamid, S. Watts, A. Fix, G. Strickland, W. Anwar, and I. Sallam. 2001. "Hepatitis C in a Community in Upper Egypt: One Cross-Sectional Survey." *Am J Trop Med Hyg* 63(5):236–41.

Nalo, D., and M. Aoko. 1994. "Macroeconomic Impact of HIV/AIDS in Kenya." Nairobi.

National AIDS Program, Iran. 2001. "AIDS in Islamic Republic of Iran." Presentation prepared for the WHO 11th Intercountry Meeting of National AIDS and STD Program Managers, Casablanca, July 2001.

National AIDS Program, Ministry of Health, Lebanon. 2002. "HIV/AIDS Prevention through Outreach to Vulnerable Groups in Beirut-Lebanon."

National AIDS Program, Ministry of Public Health, Tunisia. 2001. « Point sur la situation épidémiologique de l'infection a VIH/SIDA en Tunisie. » Processed.

National AIDS Program, Sudan. 2001. "National Program Evolution Sudan." Presentation prepared for the WHO 11th Intercountry Meeting of National AIDS and STD Program Managers, Casablanca, July 2001.

National AIDS Programme, Ministry of Health and Health Care, Jordan. 2000. "HIV Prevention for Youth in Jordan" and "HIV/AIDS and STD Prevention for Young People Outside Schools and University Settings in Jordan."

National AIDS/STD Program/Directorate General of Health Services/MOHFW/Government of the People's Republic of Bangladesh. 2001. "HIV in Bangladesh: Where Is It Going? Background document for the dissemination of the third round of national HIV and behavioral surveillance, Dhaka, November 2001.

National Research Council. 1977. "Improving Reproductive Health in Developing Countries." Population Reference Bureau.

Njoh, J., and S. Zimmo. 1997. "The Prevalence of Human Immunodeficiency Virus among Drug-Dependent Patients in Jeddah, Saudi Arabia." *J Subst Abuse Treat* 14(5):487–88.

Obermeyer, Carla M. 1994. "Reproductive Choice in Islam: Gender and State in Iran and Tunisia." *Studies in Family Planning* 25 (1):41–51.

———. 2000. "Sexuality in Morocco: Changing Context and Contested Domain." *Culture, Health, and Sexuality* 2(3):239–54.

Oelrichs, R. B., I. L. Shrestha, N. A. Anderson, and N. J. Deacon. 2000. "The Explosive Human Immunodeficiency Virus Type 1 Epidemic among Injecting Drug Users of Kathmandu, Nepal, Is Caused by a

Subtype C Virus of Restricted Genetic Diversity." *J Virology* 74:1149–57.

Omran, A., and F. Roudi. 1993. "The Middle East Population Puzzle." *Population Bulletin* 48(1).

Over, M. 1992. "The Macroeconomic Impact of AIDS in Sub-Saharan Africa." Working Paper. World Bank, Population and Human Resources Department.

———. 1997. "The Effects of Societal Variables on Urban Rates of HIV Infection in Developing Countries: An Exploratory Analysis." European Commission.

———. 1998. "Towards Estimating the Impact of AIDS on Social Welfare: A Methodological Note with an Application to Malawi." World Bank. Processed.

Over, M., P. Mujinja, D. Dorsainvil, and I. Gupta. 2001. "Impact of Adult Death on Household Expenditures in Kagera, Tanzania." Policy Research Working Paper. World Bank, Policy Research Department, Washington, D.C.

Peak, A., S. Rana, S. H. Maharjan, D. Jolley, and N. Crofts. 1995. "Declining Risk for HIV among Injecting Drug Users in Kathmandu, Nepal: The Impact of a Harm-Reduction Program." *AIDS* 9(9):1067–70.

Petro-Nustas, W. 1999. "Men's Knowledge and Attitudes towards Birth Spacing and Contraceptive Use in Jordan." *International Family Planning Perspectives* 25(4):181–85.

Philippon, M., M. Saada, M. A. Kamil, and H. M. Houmed. 1997. "Attendance at a Health Center by Clandestine Prostitutes in Djibouti." *Santé* 7(1):5–10.

Plan and Budget Organization, Tehran, and the United Nations. 1999. "Human Development Report of the Islamic Republic of Iran, 1999." Tehran.

Population Council. 1998. "Transitions to Adulthood: A National Survey of Adolescents in Egypt." Regional Office for West Asia and North Africa, Population Council, Cairo.

Preble, E. (AIDSCAP). 1996. "Needs Assessment for HIV/AIDS Control and Prevention in Egypt." Report to the U.S. Agency for International Development. Cairo. Processed.

Quattek. 2000. "The Economic Impact of AIDS in South Africa: A Dark Cloud on the Horizon." Processed.

Razzaghi, E., A. Rahimi, M. Hosseni, S. Madani, and A. Chatterjee. 1999. "Rapid Situation Assessment (RSA) of Drug Abuse in Iran." Short version of the English report. Prevention Department, State Welfare Organization Ministry of Health, Tehran, and Joint United Nations Drug Control Programme. Processed.

Rehle, T., T. Saidel, S. Hassig, P. Bouey, E. Gaillard, and D. Sokal. 1998. "AVERT: A User-Friendly Model to Estimate the Impact of HIV/Sexually Transmitted Disease Prevention Interventions on HIV Transmission." *AIDS* 12 (Suppl 2):S27–S35.

Renaud, M. 1997. *Women at the Crossroads: A Prostitute Community's Response to AIDS in Urban Senegal.* United Kingdom: Gordon and Breach.

Renganathan, E., I. Quinti, E. El Ghazzawi, O. Kader, I. El Sherbini, F. Gamil, and G. Rocchi. 1995. "Absence of HIV-1 and HIV-2 Infection in Different Populations from Alexandria, Egypt." *Eur J Epidemiol* 11(6):711–12.

Republic of Yemen and United Nations Development Programme. 1998. "Yemen Human Development Report 1998." Republic of Yemen Ministry of Planning and Development, Sana'a.

République Algérienne Démocratique et Populaire Ministère de la Santé et de la Population/Direction de la Prévention/Institut National de Santé Publique. 2000. « Premier séminaire d'information et d'évaluation du projet PNUD/Gouvernement ALG/94/010. » Surveillance des Risques de Santé Liés à la Route Transsaharienne. Processed.

Reuters New Service. 2001a. "Bahrain Visa Curbs Only on Women from CIS States." May 1, 2001.

———. 2001b. "Iran Arrests Members of Sex Trade Ring." Tehran, August 1, 2001.

Reysoo, F. 1999. "Gender, Reproductive Rights, and Health in Morocco: Traps for Unmarried Mothers." *Development* 42(1):63–66.

Ridanovic, Z. 1997. "AIDS and Islam." *Med Arh* 51(1–2):45–46.

Riyad, M., N. Trombati, A. Benschekroune, B. Charaf, A. Nabaoui, Z. Bouayad, and A. Benslimane. 1992. "HIV Infection among Tuberculous Patients in Morocco." *Eur Respir J* 5(5):642.

Robalino, D., A. Voetberg, and O. Picaso. 2002. "The Macroeconomic Impacts of HIV/AIDS in Kenya: Estimating Optimal Reduction Targets for the HIV Incidence Rate." *Journal of Policy Modeling* 24:195–218.

Rodier, G., E. Fox, N. T. Constantine, and E. A. Abbatte. 1990. "HHV-6 in Djibouti—an Epidemiological Survey in Young Adults." *Trans R Soc Trop Med Hyg* 84(1).

Rodier, G., B. Couzineau, S. Salah, J. Bouloumie, J. P. Parra, E. Fox, N. Constantine, and D. Watts. 1993a. "Infection by the Human Immunodeficiency Virus in the Republic of Djibouti: Literature Review and Regional Data." *Med Trop (Mars)* 53(1):61–67.

Rodier, G. R., B. Couzineau, G. C. Gray, C. S. Omar, E. Fox, J. Bouloumie, and D. Watts. 1993b. "Trends of Human Immunodeficiency Virus Type-1 Infection in Female Prostitutes and Males Diagnosed with a Sexually Transmitted Disease in Djibouti, East Africa." *Am J Trop Med Hyg* 48(5):682–86.

Rodier, G. R., J. J. Morand, J. S. Olson, D. M. Watts, and Said-Salah. 1993c. "HIV Infection among Secondary School Students in Djibouti, Horn of Africa: Knowledge, Exposure, and Prevalence." *East Africa Med J* 70(7):414–17.

Rodier, G. R., J. P. Sevre, G. Binson, G. C. Gray, Said-Salah, and P. Gravier. 1993d. "Clinical Features Associated with HIV-1 Infection in Adult Patients Diagnosed with Tuberculosis in Djibouti, Horn of Africa." *Trans R Soc Trop Med Hyg* 87(6):676–77.

Rosa, B. 1999. « Serosurveillance épidémiologique de l'infection au VIH par réseau sentinelle. » Université d'Alger, Faculté de Médecine d'Alger, Département de Médecine, thèse de DESM.

Ruggi, Suzanne. 2000. "Commodifying Honor in Female Sexuality: Honor Killings in Palestine." In Pinar Ilkkaracen, ed., *Women and Sexuality in Muslim Societies*, pp. 393–98. Istanbul: Women for Women's Human Rights/Kaddinin Insan Haklari Projesi.

Ryan, C. A., A. Zidouh, L. E. Manhart, R. Selka, M. Xia, M. Moloney-Kitts, J. Mahjour, M. Krone, B. N. Courtois, G. Dallabetta, and K. K. Holmes. 1998. "Reproductive Tract Infections in Primary Health Care, Family Planning, and Dermatovenereology Clinics: Evaluation of Syndromic Management in Morocco." *Sex Transm Infect* 74(Suppl 1):S95–S105.

Saidel, T., D. Des Jarlais, W. Peerapatanapokin, J. Dorabjee, S. Singh, and T. Brown. 2003. "Potential Impact of HIV among IDUs on Heterosexual Transmission in Asian Settings: Scenarios from the Asian Epidemic Model." *International Journal of Drug Policy* 14:63–74.

Saleh, M. A., Y. S. al-Ghamdi, O. A. al-Yahia, T. M. Shaqran, and A. R. Mosa. 2000. "Impact of Health Education Programs on Knowledge about AIDS and HIV Transmission in Students of Secondary Schools in Buraidah City, Saudi Arabia: An Exploratory Study." *East Mediter Health J* 5(5):1068–75.

Salem, A. 1992. "A Condom Sense Approach to AIDS Prevention: A Historical Perspective." *S D J Med* 45(10):294–96.

Schmitt, A., and J. Sofer, eds. 1992. *Sexuality and Eroticism among Males in Moslem Societies*. New York: Harrington Park Press/Haworth Press.

Schuler, S. R., S. M. Hashemi, A. P. Riley, and S. Akhter. 1996. "Credit Programs, Patriarchy, and Men's Violence against Women in Rural Bangladesh." *Soc Sci Med* 43(12):1729–42.

Seif El Dawla, A., A. Abdel Hadi, and N. Abdel Wahab. 1998. "Women's Wit over Men's: Trade-Offs and Strategic Accommodations in Egyptian Women's Reproductive Lives." In R. Petchesky and K. Judd, eds., *Negotiating Reproductive Rights: Women's Perspectives across Countries and Cultures*, pp. 69–107. Atlantic Highlands, N.J.: Zed Books.

Shaaban, Bouthaina. 1998. "Persisting Contradictions: Muslim Women in Syria." In Herbert L. Bodman and Nayereh Tohidi, eds., *Women in Muslim Societies: Diversity within Unity*, pp. 101–17. Boulder, Colo.: Lynne Rienner Publishers.

———. 2000. "Love and Life at Al Tawariqu Society." In Pinar Ilkkaracen, ed., *Women and Sexuality in Muslim Societies*, pp. 171–86. Istanbul:
Women for Women's Human Rights/Kaddinin Insan Haklari Projesi.

Shah, Nasra M., Makhdoom A. Shah, and Zoran Radovanovic. 1998.
"Patterns of Desired Fertility and Contraceptive Use in Kuwait." *International Family Planning Perspectives* 24(3):133–38.

Shanks, N. J., and D. al-Kalai. 1995. "Occupation Risk of Needlestick
Injuries among Health Care Personnel in Saudi Arabia." *J Hosp Infect*
29(3):221–26.

Sheba, M. F., J. N. Woody, A. M. Zaki, J. C. Morrill, J. Burans, I. Farag,
S. Kashaba, S. Madkour, and M. Mansour. 1988. "The Prevalence of
HIV Infection in Egypt." *Trans R Soc Trop Med Hyg* 82(4):634.

Shokrollahi, P., M. Mirmohamadi, F. Mehrabi, and G. H. Babaei. 1999.
"Prevalence of Sexual Dysfunction in Women Seeking Services at
Family Planning Centers in Tehran." *Journal of Sex and Marital Ther-
apy* 25(3):211–15.

Slama, J., N. Mojaat, M. Bjaoui, F. Durant, D. Gueguen, K. Boukef, and
B. Genetet. 1992. "Prevalence of Hepatitis C in Multitransfused
Tunisian Patients." *Nouv Rev Fr Hematol* 34(4):301-02.

Sonbol, Amira. 2000. "Rape and Law in Ottoman and Modern Egypt."
In Pinar Ilkkaracen, ed., *Women and Sexuality in Muslim Societies*, pp.
309–26. Istanbul: Women for Women's Human Rights/Kaddinin
Insan Haklari Projesi.

Soueif, Moustafa. 1994. "Extent and Patterns of Drug Use among Students and Working-Class Men in Egypt." National Center for Social
and Criminological Research, Cairo. Processed.

Sow, A. 2001. "HIV/AIDS Epidemic and Sexually Transmitted Diseases
in Djibouti Republic." Prepared for the WHO 11th Intercountry
Meeting of National AIDS and STD Program Managers, Casablanca,
July 2001.

Stevenson, T. B. 1997. "Migration, Family, and Household in Highland
Yemen: The Impact of Socio-Economic and Political Change and
Cultural Ideals on Domestic Organization." *J Comparative Family
Studies* 28(2):14–53.

Stover, J. 1997. "The Future Demographic Impacts of AIDS: What Do We Know?" World Bank.

Stover, John, and Peter Way. 1995. "Impact of Interventions on Reducing the Spread of HIV in Africa: Computer Simulations Applications." *African Medical Practice* 2(4).

Sudan National AIDS Control Program. 2000. "HIV/AIDS/STD Surveillance Report, Third Quarter Report, 2000." Khartoum.

———. 2001. "HIV/AIDS/STI Surveillance Report, First Quarter Report, 2001." Khartoum.

Sudan National AIDS Control Program, Federal MOH. 2002. "Report Situation Analysis: Behavioural and Epidemiological Surveys and Response Analysis." Khartoum.

Sultanate of Oman, HIV/AIDS/STI Prevention and Control Program, Department of Surveillance and Disease Control, Directorate-General of Health Affairs, Ministry of Health. 2001. "HIV/AIDS and STI Prevention through Peer Education among Young People in the Sultanate of Oman." UNAIDS Activity Proposal. Processed.

Sweat, M., and J. Denison. 1995. "Reducing HIV in Developing Countries with Structural and Environmental Interventions." *AIDS* 9 (Suppl A):S251–57.

Syrian Arab Republic. 2001a. "Country Report." Prepared for the WHO 11th Intercountry Meeting of National AIDS and STD Program Managers, Casablanca, July 2001.

———. 2001b. "HIV/AIDS and STD Surveillance System-Syrian Arab Republic." Prepared for the WHO 11th Intercountry Meeting of National AIDS and STD Program Managers, Casablanca, July 2001.

Task Force on HIV and Vulnerability. 2000. "Drug Use and HIV Vulnerability Policy: Research Study in Asia (October 2000)." Joint United Nations Programme on HIV/AIDS/United Nations Drug Control Programme, Bangkok.

Tastemain, C., and P. Coles. 1993. "Can a Culture Stop AIDS in its Tracks?" *New Scientist* (September) 11:13-14.

Tawil, O., K. O'Reilly, I. Coulibaly, A. Tiémélé, H. Himmich, A. Boushaba, K. Pradeep, and M. Caraël. 1999. "HIV Prevention among Vulnerable Populations: Outreach in the Developing World." *AIDS* 13(Suppl A): S239–47.

Tchupo, Jean Paul. 1998. « Rapport de mission. Les maladies sexuellement transmissibles en République de Djibouti: Evaluation de la situation et recommandations pour une prise en charge optimale. » Joint United Nations Programme on HIV/AIDS. Processed.

The Economist. 2001. "Sex Bomb: AIDS in Asia." October 6–12, p. 34.

The Living Non-Related Renal Transplant Study Group. 1997. "Commercially Motivated Renal Transplantation: Results in 540 Patients Transplanted in India." *Clin Transplant* 11(6):536–44.

Tiouiri, H., B. Louzir, N. Ben Salem, M. Beji, B. Kilani, M. Gastli, J. Daghfous, and A. Zribi. 1995. "Standard Radiological Characteristics of Thoracic Sites of Tuberculosis in Patients with AIDS in a Tunisian Population." *Rev Pneumol Clin* 51(6):321–24.

Tiouiri, H., B. Naddari, G. Khiari, S. Hajjem, and A. Zribi. 2000. "Study of Psychosocial Factors in HIV-Infected Patients in Tunisia." *East Mediterranean Health J* 5(5):903–11.

Toufic, A. 1996–97. « Pratiques et mobilité des usagers de drogues: de la dynamique du risque a celle de prevention. » *Le Journal du Sida* (numéro special: Monde Arabe, Migrants/Maghreb) 92–93:31–36.

Tunisian External Communication Agency/National Union of Tunisian Women. 1993. *Women of Tunisia: Their Struggle and Their Gains.* Tunisian External Communication Agency. (Popline).

UNAIDS (Joint United Nations Programme on HIV/AIDS). 1999. "Project Proposal: Development of Policy and Strategies in Care and Support for People Living with HIV/AIDS." Yemen.

———. 2000. "HIV Situation and Needs Assessment: Project on Development of Policy and Strategies in Care and Support for People Living with HIV/AIDS." Yemen. Processed.

———. 2001a. "Report of the Regional Meeting of UNAIDS Cosponsors and Key Partners." Cairo.

———. 2001b. "The Global Strategy Framework on HIV/AIDS."

UNAIDS/MENA (Joint United Nations Programme on HIV/AIDS/Middle East and North Africa). 2000. "HIV/AIDS in the Middle East and North Africa: Strategic Objectives for 2000–2001." Processed.

UNAIDS/WHO (Joint United Nations Programme on HIV/AIDS/World Health Organization). 2000a. "Guidelines for Second Generation HIV Surveillance." Geneva.

———. 2000b. "Kenya Epidemiological Fact Sheet on HIV/AIDS and Sexually Transmitted Infections." Geneva.

———. 2001. "AIDS Epidemic Update." Geneva.

———. 2002a. "AIDS Epidemic Update." Geneva.

———. 2002b. "Algeria Epidemiological Fact Sheet on HIV/AIDS and Sexually Transmitted Infections." Geneva.

———. 2002c. "Bahrain Epidemiological Fact Sheet on HIV/AIDS and Sexually Transmitted Infections." Geneva.

———. 2002d. "Djibouti Epidemiological Fact Sheet on HIV/AIDS and Sexually Transmitted Infections." Geneva.

———. 2002e. "Egypt Epidemiological Fact Sheet on HIV/AIDS and Sexually Transmitted Infections." Geneva.

———. 2002f. "Ethiopia Epidemiological Fact Sheet on HIV/AIDS and Sexually Transmitted Infections." Geneva.

———. 2002g. "Islamic Republic of Iran Epidemiological Fact Sheet on HIV/AIDS and Sexually Transmitted Infections." Geneva.

———. 2002h. "Jordan Epidemiological Fact Sheet on HIV/AIDS and Sexually Transmitted Infections." Geneva.

———. 2002i. "Kuwait Epidemiological Fact Sheet on HIV/AIDS and Sexually Transmitted Infections." Geneva.

———. 2002j. "Lebanon Epidemiological Fact Sheet on HIV/AIDS and Sexually Transmitted Infections." Geneva.

———. 2002k. "Libya Epidemiological Fact Sheet on HIV/AIDS and Sexually Transmitted Infections." Geneva.

———. 2002l. "Morocco Epidemiological Fact Sheet on HIV/AIDS and Sexually Transmitted Infections." Geneva.

———. 2002m. "Oman Epidemiological Fact Sheet on HIV/AIDS and Sexually Transmitted Infections." Geneva.

———. 2002n. "Qatar Epidemiological Fact Sheet on HIV/AIDS and Sexually Transmitted Infections." Geneva.

———. 2002o. "Saudi Arabia Epidemiological Fact Sheet on HIV/AIDS and Sexually Transmitted Infections." Geneva.

———. 2002p. "Sudan Epidemiological Fact Sheet on HIV/AIDS and Sexually Transmitted Infections." Geneva.

———. 2002q. "Syria Epidemiological Fact Sheet on HIV/AIDS and Sexually Transmitted Infections." Geneva.

———. 2002r. "Tunisia Epidemiological Fact Sheet on HIV/AIDS and Sexually Transmitted Infections." Geneva.

———. 2002s. "United Arab Emirates Epidemiological Fact Sheet on HIV/AIDS and Sexually Transmitted Infections." Geneva.

———. 2002t. "Yemen Epidemiological Fact Sheet on HIV/AIDS and Sexually Transmitted Infections." Geneva.

UNDP (United Nations Development Programme). 2000. "Formulation of the National Policy Framework to Control the Spread of HIV/AIDS in Yemen." Project of the government of Yemen.

———. 2001. *Human Development Report 2000*. New York and Oxford: Oxford University Press.

UNESCO/UNAIDS (United Nations Educational, Scientific, and Cultural Organization/Joint United Nations Programme on HIV/AIDS). 2001. "Regional Seminar on Integration of HIV/AIDS within the School System," Brumana, Lebanon, October 1–5, 2001.

UNFPA (United Nations Population Fund). 2000. "Strategic Partnership with the Arab Scout Organization for Youth Reproductive Health." Briefing paper. Tunisia. Processed.

UNHCR (United Nations High Commissioner for Refugees). 1999. "Djibouti." (Web).

———. 2001. "Recent Developments, East and Horn of Africa. 2001 Global Appeal."

UNICEF (United Nations Children's Fund). 2001a. *The State of the World's Children 2001. Early Childhood*. New York.

———. 2001b. "Early Marriage: Child Spouses." *Innocenti Digest* 7. Florence.

United Arab Emirates. 2001. "UAE's National Program for AIDS Control and Prevention." Prepared for the WHO 11th Intercountry Meeting of National AIDS and STD Program Managers, Casablanca, July 2001.

United Nations. 2001. "Yemen Common Country Assessment." United Nations in Yemen.

UNODC (United Nations Office on Drugs and Crime). 2003. Middle East Programme, http://www.unodc.org/pdf/middle_east_programme.pdf (accessed April 25, 2003).

UNODCCP (United Nations Office of Drug Control and Crime Prevention). 2000a. "Algeria: Overview of Drug Control Situation." (Web).

———. 2000b. "Egypt: Overview of Drug Control Situation." (Web).

——— 2000c. "Jordan: Overview of Drug Control Situation." (Web).

———. 2000d. "Libya: Overview of Drug Control Situation." (Web).

———. 2000e. "Oman: Overview of Drug Control Situation." (Web).

———. 2000f. "Syria: Overview of Drug Control Situation." (Web).

———. 2000g. "Tunisia: Overview of Drug Control Situation." (Web).

———. 2000h. "Djibouti: Country Profile." Kenya Regional Office. (Web).

———. 2001a. "Islamic Republic of Iran. Country Profile." (Web).

———. 2001b. "Rapid Assessment of Trends and Patterns of Drug Abuse in Egypt." Final Report. UNODCCP/Ministry of Health, Cairo.

———. 2001c. "Illicit Drug Markets in Greater Cairo." Cairo.

USAID (United States Agency for International Development)/Egypt. 2001a. "Briefing Background." Cairo. Processed.

———. 2001b. "Situation Analysis: HIV/AIDS." Briefing Paper. Processed.

U.S. Census Bureau. 1997. "Recent HIV Seroprevalence Levels by Country: January 1997." Research Note 23. Health Studies Branch, International Programs Center, Population Division, Washington, D.C.

———. 2001. "Monitoring the Epidemic (MAP): The Status and Trends of HIV/AIDS/STI Epidemics in Asia and the Pacific." Melbourne, Australia.

U.S. State Department (NEA/ARP and PRM/POP). 2001. "HIV-AIDS Event Draws Large Turnout." Unclassified cable, E.O. 12958, February 26, 2001.

Voevodin, A., K. A. Crandall, P. Seth, and S. al Mufti. 1996. "HIV Type 1 Subtypes B and C from New Regions of India and Indian and Ethiopian Expatriates in Kuwait." *AIDS Res Hum Retroviruses* 12(7):641–43.

Von Bruck, Gabrielle. 1997. "Elusive Bodies: The Politics of Aesthetics among Yemeni Elite Women." *Signs* 23(1):175–214.

Walker, N., J. M. Garcia-Calleja, L. Heaton, E. Asamoah-Odei, G. Poumeral, S. Lazzari, P. Ghys, B. Schwartländer, and K. Stanecki. 2001. "Epidemiological Analysis of the Quality of HIV Sero-Surveillance in the World: How Well Do We Track the Epidemic?" *AIDS* 15:1545–54.

Watts, D. M., N. T. Constantine, M. F. Sheba, M. Kamal, J. Callahan, and M. E. Kilpatrick. 1993. "Prevalence of HIV Infection and AIDS in Egypt over Four Years of Surveillance (1986–1990)." *J Trop Med Hyg* 96(2):113–17.

Whitaker, B. 2000. "Girl Killed to Act as Drug Mule in Gulf." *The Guardian*, May 10, 2000.

WHO (World Health Organization). 1991. "Global Program on AIDS." Global HIV/AIDS Estimates and Projections Update. SFI/RES/GPA/HQ.

———. 2000. "The World Health Report 2000. Health Systems: Improving Performance." Geneva.

———. 2001. "Global AIDS Surveillance." *Weekly Epidemiological Record* 50(76):389–400.

WHO/EMRO (World Health Organization/Eastern Mediterranean Office). 1995. "Report on the Intercountry Workshop on Evaluation of National AIDS Programs." Nicosia, Cyprus, August 22–25, 1995. WHO-EM/GPA/111/E. Processed.

———. 1999. "Report on the Intercountry Consultation for Development of Guidelines for Demand Reduction in Substance Abuse with Special Emphasis on Injecting Drug Use." WHO-EM/MNH/156/E/L. Beirut, November 25–27, 1999. Processed.

———. 2000a. "Regional Consultation on Reducing Risk and Vulnerability to HIV/AIDS in Countries of the Eastern Mediterranean Region." Tunis, Tunisia, May 29–June 1, 2000.

———. 2000b. "Global and Regional HIV Situation, 2000." EM/RC47/Inf. Doc. 2. Processed.

———. 2000c. "Somalia: Country Brief." Updated on November 28, 2000.

———. 2000d. "The RD Report 2000, AIDS and Sexually Transmitted Diseases." Processed.

———. 2001a. "Progress Report. Acquired Immunodeficiency Syndrome (AIDS) in the Eastern Mediterranean Region." EM/RC48/Inf. Doc. 2. Processed.

———. 2001b. "Report on the Regional Consultation to Strengthen STD Prevention and Care Strategies in the Countries of the Eastern Mediterranean." Cairo, May 7–10, 2001. Processed.

———. 2001c. "Report on the Regional Consultation towards Improving HIV/AIDS and STD Surveillance in the Countries of the Eastern Mediterranean Region." Beirut, Lebanon, October 30–November 2, 2000. Processed.

———. 2001d. "Sudan: Country Brief." Updated on May 3, 2001.

———. 2003. "Regional Meeting on Expanded Access to HIV/AIDS Treatment in the Countries of the EMR." Cairo, February 18–20, 2003.

WHO/EMRO and UNAIDS. 2001. "Assessment of the HIV/AIDS and STD Situation and Response in the Sultanate of Oman." February 17–25, 2001.

Wikan, Unni. 1976. "Man Becomes Woman—Transvestism in Oman." *Tisskrift for samfunnsforskning* 17(4):318–34. (Popline).

World Bank. 1993. "Staff Appraisal Report." Report 11900-YEM. Republic of Yemen Family Health Project.

———. 1997a. "Country Assistance Strategy for the Republic of Lebanon." Report 17153.

———. 1997b. "Djibouti: Crossroads of the Horn of Africa Poverty Assessment." Report 16543-DJI. Human Development Group IV, Africa Region, Washington, D.C.

———. 1998a. "Health, Nutrition, and Population in Middle East and North Africa Region: Background Paper for the Regional Seminar on Health Sector Development in Middle East and North Africa."

———. 1998b. "Project Appraisal Document for a Proposed Loan in an Amount Equal to FRF 297,600,000 to the Republic of Tunisia for a Health Sector Loan, Feb 13, 1998." MENA Report 17358-TUN. Human Development Sector.

———. 1999a. *Confronting AIDS: Public Priorities in a Global Epidemic.* New York: Oxford University Press, 1997; revised edition, 1999.

———. 1999b. "Country Assistance Strategy for the Republic of Jordan." Report 19890.

———. 1999c. "Country Assistance Strategy for the Republic of Yemen." Report 19073.

———. 1999d. "Project Appraisal Document for a Proposed Loan in an Amount Equal to US$35.0 Million to the Hashemite Kingdom of Jordan for a Health Sector Reform Project, March 5, 1999." MENA Report #19006-JO. Human Development Sector.

———. 2000a. "Algeria at a Glance." (Web).

———. 2000b. "Bahrain at a Glance." (Web).

———. 2000c. "Country Assistance Strategy for the Republic of Tunisia." Report 20161.

———. 2000d. "Cultural Heritage Building Block [Yemen]." Infrastructure Development Group, Middle East and North Africa Region.

———. 2000e. "Egypt, Arab Republic at a Glance." (Web).

———. 2000f. "Middle East and North Africa." In *World Bank Annual Report 2000*, pp. 74–79. Washington, D.C.

———. 2000g. "Project Appraisal Document on a Proposed Credit in the Amount of SDR 11.4 (US$15.0 million) to the Republic of Djibouti for the International Road Corridor Rehabilitation Project." Report 20365-DJI.

———. 2000h. "Project Appraisal Document for a Proposed Loan in an Amount Equal to US$87.0 Million to the Islamic Republic of Iran for a Second Primary Health Care and Nutrition Project, April 3, 2000." MENA Report 20202-IRN. Human Development Group.

———. 2000i. "Project Appraisal Document on a Proposed Credit in the Amount of SDR 56 Million (US$75 Million Equivalent) to the Republic of Yemen for a Second Social Fund for Development Project, April 11, 2000."

———. 2000j. "Republic of Yemen. Comprehensive Development Review." Building Block on Education.

———. 2000k. "Republic of Yemen. Comprehensive Development Review." Building Block on Urbanization.

———. 2000l. "Republic of Yemen. Comprehensive Development Review." Health Sector Phase I. Processed.

———. 2000m. "Republic of Yemen. Comprehensive Development Review Phase I, Judicial and Legal System Building Block." Legal Department.

———. 2000n. "Republic of Yemen. Comprehensive Development Review Phase I, Poverty and Social Safety Nets Building Block." Social and Economic Development Unit, Middle East and North Africa Region.

———. 2000o. "The World Bank and Yemen: Country Brief." (Web).

———. 2001a. "A Framework for Social Protection in the MENA Region." Washington, D.C.

———. 2001b. "Country Assistance Strategy for the Republic of Egypt." Report 22163.

———. 2001c. "Country Assistance Strategy for the Republic of Iran." Report 22050.

———. 2001d. "Country Assistance Strategy for the Kingdom of Morocco." Report 22115.

———. 2001e. "Islamic Republic of Iran. Expanded Program for Immunization in the New Millennium: Lessons Learned."

———. 2001f. "Reducing Vulnerability and Increasing Opportunity: Social Protection in the Middle East and North Africa." Orientations in Development Series. Middle East and North Africa Region. Washington, D.C.

———. 2001g. "Regional Update." MENA. Available at http://worldbank.org/UNGASS/MENA.htm.

———. 2002a. "Algeria Public Expenditures Review in the Social Sectors." Report 22591-AL.

———. 2002b. World Development Indicators Database (SIMA).

———. Report #20291-YEM. Human Development Sector, MENA Region.

World Bank Group. 2000a. "Djibouti Macroeconomic Brief." (Web).

———. 2000b. "Egypt in Brief." (Web).

———. 2000c. "Middle East and North Africa Data Profile." World Development Indicators Database. (Web).

———. 2000d. "Yemen Republic, Data Profile." World Development Indicators Database. (Web).

———. 2001. "Algeria in Brief." (Web).

World Bank Memorandum. 1990. "Project Completion Report on Republic of Tunisia Health and Population Project (Loan 2005-Tun)."

———. 2001. "Country Assistance Strategy for the Republic of Djibouti." Report 21414-DJI.

Yeghaneh, Bahram. 2001. Presentation on HIV/AIDS in Iran, at MAP Meeting, Melbourne, Australia, October 4, 2001.

Yerly, S., R. Quadri, F. Negro, K. Posfay Barbe, J.-J. Cheseaux, P. Burgisser, C.-A. Siegrist, and L. Perrin. 2001. "Nosocomial Outbreak of Multiple Bloodborne Viral Infections." *J Infect Dis* 184:369–72.

Yousif, A., M. Wallace, and B. Baig. 1994. "The Seroprevalence of Syphilis, Toxoplasmosis, and Hepatitis B in Patients in Bahrain Infected with Human Immunodeficiency Virus." *Trans R Soc Trop Med Hyg* 88(1):60.

Zahra, Rim. 2000. "The High Price of Walking." In Pinar Ilkkaracen ed., *Women and Sexuality in Muslim Societies*. Istanbul: Women for Women's Human Rights/Kaddinin Insan Haklari Projesi.

Zakharia, L. F., and S. Tabari. 1997. "Health, Work Opportunities, and Attitudes: A Review of Palestinian Women's Situation in Lebanon." *J Refugee Studies* 10(3):411–29.

Zawawi, T. H., M. A. Abdelaal, A. Y. Mohamed, D. J. Rowbottom, W. A. Alyafi, K. H. Marzouki, and A. A. Rashed. 1997. "Routine Preoperative Screening for Human Immunodeficiency Virus in a General Hospital, Saudi Arabia." *Infect Control Hosp Epidemiol* 18(3):158–59.

Index